Emerging Technologies and Concepts for Cardiovascular Risk Detection

This accessible guide to advanced medical technologies and methodologies for monitoring, diagnosing, and predicting cardiovascular diseases addresses sensor technologies and noninvasive monitoring methods and looks at the growing integration of machine learning and artificial intelligence (AI).

The authors guide readers from an introduction to the cardiovascular system and a review of traditional and modern diagnostic methods before explaining recent advances in medical technology, such as wearable smart devices and their sensor types (namely, pressure, photoelectric, and ultrasonic), and how these advances have been applied to cardiovascular disease diagnosis and detection. Key topics include pulse wave analysis, sensor technology for radial blood pressure monitoring, and the integration of AI to enhance predictive accuracy. With a focus on continuous monitoring solutions, this book highlights groundbreaking research on noninvasive detection methods and the development of intelligent health systems for real-time patient evaluation. The authors also discuss how the widespread implementation of machine learning and deep learning techniques have influenced the field and propose new methods for enhancing continuous monitoring and risk prediction systems. The information within this book will help to bridge the gap between research and clinical practice.

This short guide is a valuable resource primarily for academic readers in the fields of biomedical engineering, physics, computer science, and medical imaging. Clinicians will also benefit from the discussions of applications and future research and clinical trends.

Emerging Technologies and Concepts for Cardiovascular Risk Detection

Denesh Sooriamoorthy, M. B. Malarvili,
Aindi Anas, and Olivier Meste

CRC Press
Taylor & Francis Group
Boca Raton London New York

CRC Press is an imprint of the
Taylor & Francis Group, an **informa** business

First edition published 2026

by CRC Press

2385 NW Executive Center Drive, Suite 320, Boca Raton FL 33431

and by CRC Press

4 Park Square, Milton Park, Abingdon, Oxon, OX14 4RN

CRC Press is an imprint of Taylor & Francis Group, LLC

© 2026 Denesh Sooriamoorthy, M. B. Malarvili, Aindi Anas, and Olivier Meste

ISBN: 9781041047681 (hbk)

ISBN: 9781041047728 (pbk)

ISBN: 9781003629832 (ebk)

DOI: 10.1201/9781003629832

Typeset in Times

by Newgen Publishing UK

Contents

About the Authors   vii
Overview   ix

1   **Introduction**   1

2   **Cardiovascular System**   4

3   **Medical Technology**   13

4   **Diagnosing Cardiovascular Diseases**   23

5   **Cardiovascular Disease Detection and AI Integration**   30

6   **Cardiovascular System Models**   47

7   **Conclusion and Future Recommendations**   59

References   62
Index   91

About the Authors

Denesh Sooriamoorthy is a senior lecturer at Asia Pacific University of Technology & Innovation. His research focuses on cardiovascular disease detection, mechatronics, and artificial intelligence applications in healthcare. His notable publications include studies on cardiovascular risk detection, machine learning models for electric vehicle battery state estimation, and wearable biomedical technologies.

M. B. Malarvili is currently Director of Research Management Centre at Perdana University, Kuala Lumpur, and was formerly at Universiti Teknologi Malaysia (UTM). She obtained her bachelor's and master's degrees from UTM in 2001 and 2003, respectively, and her PhD from The University of Queensland, Australia, in 2007. Malarvili is actively involved in research related to medical monitoring devices that focuses on detection of neonatal seizure, sudden cardiac death, fetal heart rate monitoring, respiratory illness screening device, and many more.

Aindi Anas is a student at Polytech Grenoble specializing in information technology for health.

Olivier Meste is a professor at the Université Côte d'Azur and a researcher at the Signals and Systems Laboratory of Sophia Antipolis (I3S). He completed his PhD at the University of Nice-Sophia Antipolis in 1992.

Overview

The increasing mortality rate due to cardiovascular disease has driven researchers to develop advanced methods to support medical professionals. Although research on medical systems for monitoring and predicting cardiovascular disease is progressing, its implementation in clinical settings remains limited. This chapter reviews cardiovascular disease, traditional diagnostic approaches, and medical technologies to provide insights into recent advancements in the field. It also explores sensor selection for capturing radial blood pressure waveforms and their correlation with conventional diagnostic methods. Additionally, cardiovascular models are examined to assess heart responses without direct patient testing. Pulse wave analysis techniques for converting radial blood pressure waveforms into aortic blood pressure waveforms are discussed to improve diagnostic accuracy. The study further investigates the correlation between the converted aortic signal and cardiovascular model outputs. A literature review on machine learning and deep learning applications is conducted to establish relationships between patient signals and model parameters. Finally, an evaluation of related studies and a summary of key findings are provided, offering a comprehensive interpretation of the literature to support future research in this domain.

Introduction

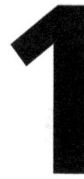

1

Cardiovascular diseases (CVDs) cause nearly 30% of mortality worldwide and may even lead to disability [1]. Approximately 17.7 million people died from CVD in 2017 [2]. This makes CVD the largest cause of death globally and one of the life-threatening diseases in most countries. It is known that total worldwide mortality caused by the various forms of CVD is approximately 2.2% or 16.7 million of the total worldwide deaths [3]. There are many forms of CVD that are avoidable by practicing prime actions on risk factors such as lack of physical activity, smoking, and unhealthy food habits [4]. Generally, the primary prevention has remained ardent to risk factor modification in the asymptomatic population [5, 6] and intervention as secondary prevention in individuals who have continual cardiovascular occurrence [7–10]. Despite all the preventions, CVD, which is a noncommunicable disease, is forecast to upsurge over the subsequent decades significantly in low- and middle-income countries [11].

In today's era with fast-paced advancement, CVD is yet the grand challenge, as it is the most dominating cause of global death, and CVD occurrences in aged people are more frequent [12]. Hence, early identification and evading illness dysfunction are critical to decreasing cardiovascular mortality by giving the concern required treatments resulting from a reliable monitoring framework. However, the early detection of CVD is typically conducted discontinuously by one-off measurement of blood pressure, Doppler ultrasonography, photoplethysmography [13], magnetic resonance imaging, and electrocardiography [14]. These methods are sole-functional, costly, intermittent, bulky, and inconvenient [15]. A self-powered, flexible wearable sensor with a miniaturized size, high sensitivity, ultralow energy consumption, and accessible usage in various scenarios is desired to monitor various cardiovascular conditions in a comfortable, continuous, real-time way and promptly discover the deterioration of cardiovascular condition [15, 16]. CVDs are multifactorial diseases resulting from a wide range of interacting environmental, social, and human factors. The current risk evaluation framework is seemingly precise by assessing patients without taking the effects of cardiovascular illness and the previously mentioned elements into thought [17].

This chapter presents a comprehensive survey on the overall topic of CVD, which relates to the technology, diagnosis, detection, and modeling. More than

DOI: 10.1201/9781003629832-1

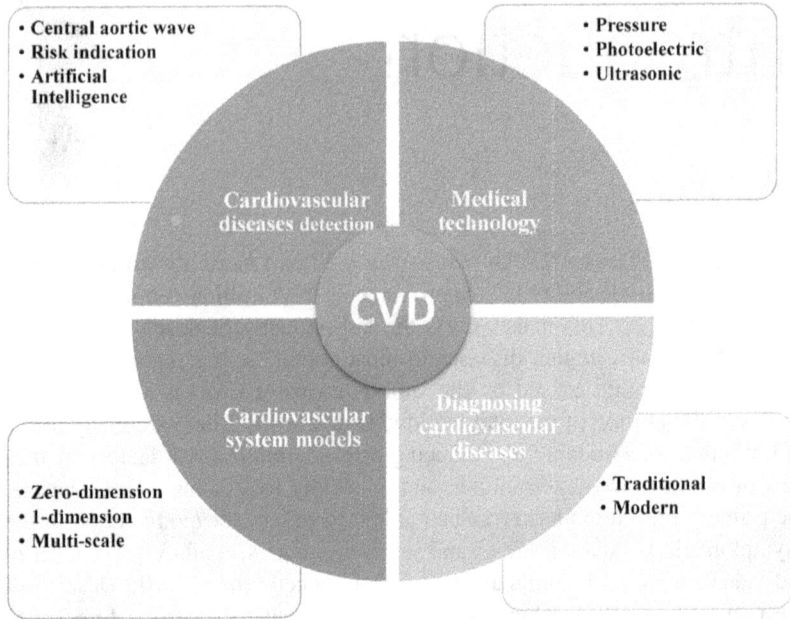

FIGURE 1.1 Categories of the survey on cardiovascular disease.

200 publications are reviewed and classified into four major categories. All these categories are further classified into two to four subcategories, which can be seen in Figure 1.1.

There are several reviews done by other researchers that address in each specific category such as medical technology [18–22], CVDs detection [23–25], and cardiovascular system models [26–29]. However, an overall review and discussion of all the categories is yet to be done, and the subcategory breakdowns are completely different compared to the other review papers. In this chapter, a review is done aimed at explaining the methods and technology that are currently used to study, detect, and monitor CVDs. This review focuses on explaining each category and discussing its interrelationship to one another. For example, medical technology is very useful in monitoring a human's heart condition, which could provide data to be analyzed. This data can be used to develop an algorithm in the detection of CVD. In addition, a preliminary study can be carried out in the cardiovascular system model to ensure that the conceptual idea on the detection of CVD is ideal. This overall approach can be related to traditional or modern methods of diagnosing. Figure 1.2 shows the number of research studies that have been carried out in each category since 2016.

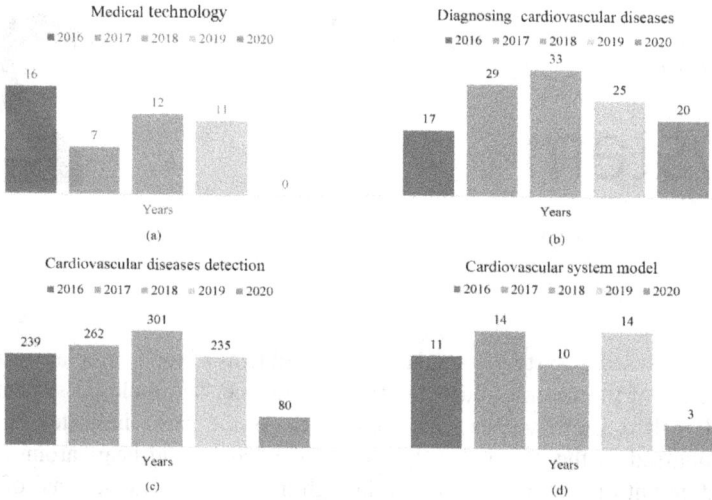

Medical technology
2016 2017 2018 2019 2020

Diagnosing cardiovascular diseases
2016 2017 2018 2019 2020

(a)

(b)

Cardiovascular diseases detection
2016 2017 2018 2019 2020

Cardiovascular system model
2016 2017 2018 2019 2020

(c)

(d)

FIGURE 1.2 The number of research studies that has been carried out in this category for the past 5 years.

This chapter is structured as follows: initially in Chapter 2, a background regarding the cardiovascular system and CVD is given. Then, Chapter 3 explains the medical technologies that are being developed for monitoring a patient's heart condition. Chapter 4 represents methods used to diagnose CVD. Chapter 5 focuses on the study of CVD and risk detection methods. Chapter 6 explains cardiovascular modeling, and Chapter 7 concludes the review of the work.

Cardiovascular System

2

The cardiovascular system is sometimes referred to as a blood vascular system. It consists of the heart, a muscular pumping device, and a closed system of vessels called arteries, veins, and capillaries. As the name indicates, blood encompassed in the circulatory system is pumped by the heart around the closed circuit of vessels as it passes through the various 'circulations' of the body [30]. This system is the body's transport system for respiratory gases, nutritive and waste materials, hormones, and heat [31]. The crucial role of the cardiovascular system in maintaining homeostasis relies on the constant and controlled movement of blood across thousands of capillaries that pervade every tissue and reach every cell in the body. It is in the microscopic capillaries that the blood carries out its ultimate transport function. Nutrients and other essential materials are transferred from capillary blood to the fluids surrounding the cells as waste products are removed [30].

2.1 THE HEART

The heart, being the center of the cardiovascular system, is a muscular organ that supplies the body with oxygen and nutrients and assists in the removal of metabolism waste via the blood vessels of the circulatory system. The heart has four chambers, and blood flows through the body. While blood is the mode of transport, the heart is the organ that keeps the blood moving through the vessels. A normal adult heart pumps about 5 liters of blood every minute. If it starts to lose its pumping efficiency for even a few minutes, the life of an individual is at risk [30]. Figure 2.1 shows the internal view of a human heart.

DOI: 10.1201/9781003629832-2

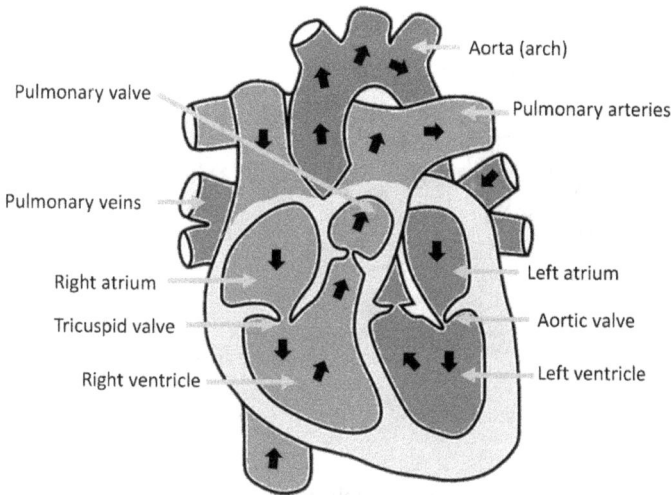

FIGURE 2.1   Internal view of the heart.

2.2 BLOOD FLOW

Blood flows through the circulation system due to continuous rhythmic contractions of the heart muscles [32]. Blood flows into the vena cava vein from all regions of the body that empties into the right atrium (RA), which collects all the deoxygenated blood. The inferior vena cava (IVC) is accountable for the collection of deoxygenated blood from the lower body, including the legs, the back, the abdomen, and the pelvis, while the superior vena cava (SVC) is responsible for collecting deoxygenated blood from the upper body, including the brain, neck, arms, and chest. All the blood collected in the RA goes directly to the right ventricle (RV), which pumps it to the main pulmonary artery and subsequently to the lungs where the blood receives fresh oxygen and releases carbon dioxide [33]. There are two components in the cardiovascular system: the pulmonary circulation and the systemic system; both are interconnected to form the circulatory system.

The circulatory system requires a particular pressure to function; this pressure is named as blood pressure. The blood pressure is divided into the systolic and diastolic blood pressures. The systolic blood pressure is measured while the heart is contracting (squeezing). When the heart contracts, the pressure in the arteries and veins rises as well. This is the upper number on a

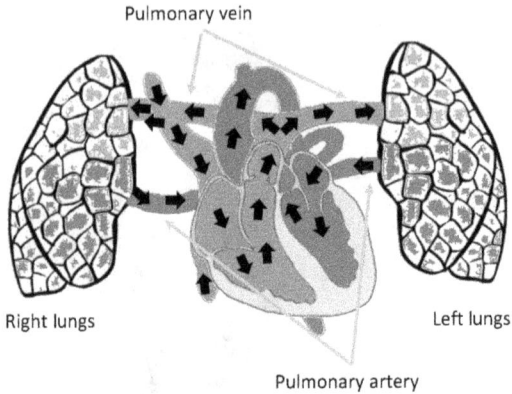

FIGURE 2.2 Pulmonary circulation.

blood pressure reading; the lower number is the diastolic blood pressure. The diastolic blood pressure is measured while the heart muscle is relaxing, also causing the pressure in the blood vessels to decrease [34].

The pulmonary circulation is responsible for the exchange of carbon dioxide for oxygen, such that oxygen-rich blood can flow throughout the body. Veins are responsible for bringing deoxygenated blood back to the heart so that this process can take place. When returning to the heart, many small veins throughout the body merge into two large veins: SVC and IVC. The IVC drains blood from below the diaphragm (the lower body), and the SVC drains blood from above the diaphragm (the upper body). Both the SVC and IVC deliver deoxygenated blood back into the RA of the heart. From the RA, blood flows through the tricuspid valve into the RV and further through the pulmonary valve into the pulmonary arteries. The blood is then carried to the lungs, where CO_2 is released, and oxygen is collected. The newly oxygenated blood travels via the pulmonary veins back to the left side of the heart [34]. The blood flow in the pulmonary circulation is shown in Figure 2.2.

The systemic circulation shown in Figure 2.3 begins within the left atrium (LA) of the heart, where newly oxygenized blood has just arrived from the lungs. The blood flows from the LA through the mitral valve into the left ventricle (LV). The LV then pumps blood through the aortic valve into the aorta (the main artery of the body), which sends the oxygen-rich blood to the body. The aorta has many branches, which give way to smaller vessels called arteries and even smaller vessels known as arterioles. This network of vessels delivers blood all throughout the body and allows for the exchange of oxygen and other nutrients within the capillary network (the connection between the arterial and venous systems). After this exchange takes place, the blood is once again

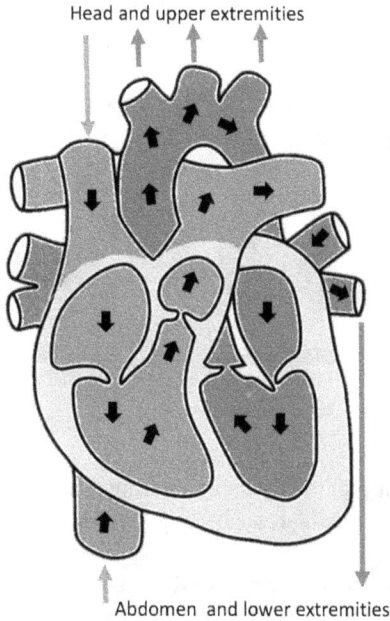

FIGURE 2.3 Systemic circulation.

oxygen-poor (but rich in carbon dioxide). It is transported via venules (the venous counterpart to arterioles) and veins (the venous counterpart to arteries) into the SVC or IVC, where the blood again enters the pulmonary circulation to become oxygenated.

2.3 CARDIAC CYCLE

The cardiac cycle shown in Figure 2.4 relates to the alternating contraction and relaxation of the myocardium in the walls of the heart chambers, coordinated by the conduction system, during a single heartbeat. Systole is the phase of contraction of the cardiac cycle, and diastole is the phase of relaxation. At normal heart rate, one cardiac cycle lasts 0.8 seconds [4]. Diastole is the period of time when the ventricles are relaxed (not contracted). Over this period, blood flows passively from the LA and the RA to the LV and the RV respectively. Blood flows through atrioventricular valves (mitral and tricuspid), which separate the atria from the ventricles. The RA receives venous blood from the body through the SVC and the IVC. The LA receives oxygenated blood from

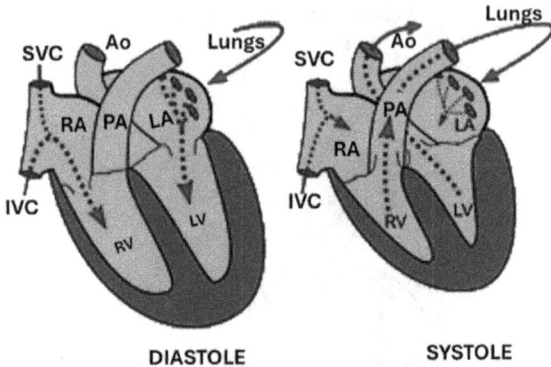

FIGURE 2.4 Cardiac cycle.

the lungs through four pulmonary veins entering the LA. At the end of the diastole, both atria contract, which pushes an additional amount of blood to the ventricles [35].

Systole indicates the time during which the LVs and RVs contract and release blood into the aorta and the pulmonary artery, respectively. During systole, the aortic and pulmonary valves are opened to allow the aorta and pulmonary artery to be ejected. The atrioventricular valves are closed during systole; therefore, no blood enters the ventricles; however, the blood continues to enter the atria through the vena cava and the pulmonary veins [35].

2.4 CARDIOVASCULAR DISEASE

CVD continues to be the dominant cause of demise worldwide, resulting in deaths that are higher than 17.3 million per year [36]. A study conducted by The Global Burden of Disease in 2010 concludes that 29.6% of all deaths globally were caused by CVD [37], and the percentage increased to 31% in 2013 [36]. Studies also show that CVDs show higher mortality than all forms of cancer combined [36]. An estimated 17 million people died from CVD in 2005, which represents 30% of all global deaths, reported by the World Health Organization (WHO). The WHO also estimates that the number could increase to 23.6 million by the year 2030 if the current trend remains [38], where it incorporates coronary heart disease (CHD), cerebrovascular disease, and arterial disease. Figure 2.5 shows the graphical representation of the major cause of deaths.

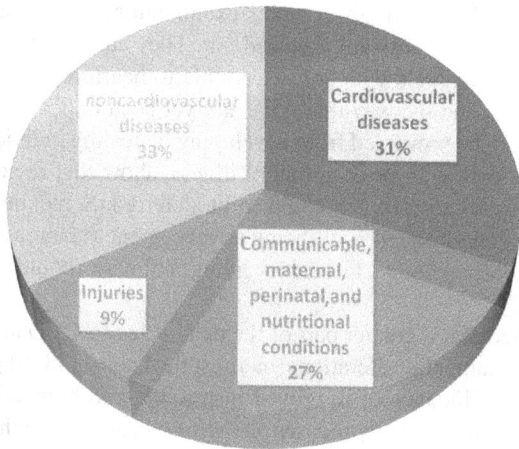

FIGURE 2.5 Major causes of death.

In addition, CVD includes several conditions that affect the heart and vasculature [39]. This may also include those influencing the blood vessels, for example, coronary artery, peripheral artery, or cerebrovascular infection, just as a heart-related disorder that can prompt raised circulatory strain, irregular heartbeat, or chest pain brought about by diminished bloodstream, among numerous others. The basic reason for diminished blood flow is the development of atherosclerotic plaque, which brings about the narrowing of veins and confines blood flow [40]. This expansion is related to an increase in smoking and dietary changes provoking an addition in serum cholesterol levels [41, 42]. The chronic CVD can hasten into a solitary horrible mishap whenever it is left untreated, for example, myocardial infarction or stroke, the two of which are related to high death rates [43–46]. Moreover, CHD and cerebrovascular disease were the first and second reasons for demise in 2016, with a rise of 39.6% and 23.8% individually since 2005 [18]. According to the National Cardiovascular Disease-Acute Coronary Syndrome (NCVD-ACS) Registry for 2011–2013, 96.8% of patients had at least one cardiovascular hazard factor, for example, hypertension. These risk factors have been on an expanding pattern. This information is not astounding as the numbers of undiagnosed and inadequately controlled hypercholesterolemia are so high [47].

Additionally, the capacity to determine acute myocardial infarction with the guide of the electrocardiogram expanded the acknowledgment of CHD before demise. While epidemiological studies have demonstrated that it is possible to reliably identify groups within the healthy population who are at an increased risk of developing ischemic heart disease, predicting this risk for an individual is not synonymous with making a pre-symptomatic diagnosis.

Screening tests and increasingly complex examinations for the early detection of ischemic coronary illness are sketched out. They can be depended upon to distinguish the individuals who are susceptible to heart disease in the future. These constraints, and the way that it has not yet been indicated that myocardial infarction can be prevented from developing in healthy individuals or from recurring in patients with prior coronary illness, show that reviews to reveal occult ischemic coronary illness ought to be deferred. Screening in essential primary settings and frequent well-being advancement to increase community awareness and responsibility to healthy living and care should be constantly emphasized [47].

It is accepted that a greater part of the deaths due to CVD are totally preventable by fundamental alterations in lifestyle habits [48–51]. While this underlines the significance of improved instruction and huge scope counteraction activities, it additionally focuses on the significance of having successful methods for distinguishing indications of ailment in the clinic, especially at an early stage [51–53]. Sustainable human development is strongly influenced by CVD, which is one of the major reasons for mortality in the world [54]. Up to 422.7 million and 17.92 million people died of CVD all over the world in 2015 [55]. It is highly recommended in clinical practice to screen in a high-risk population and early intervention of CVD [56]. The challenges of prediction and evaluation of potential CVD remain unsolved despite a lot of effort taken by the medical community [56]. Research shows that cardiovascular coincidences occur at uneven distribution during the 24 hours of the day [57] and have a high tendency to occur during the wakefulness sleep instead of later in the day [58]. However, the reason for the increase in cardiovascular occurrences in the morning is still unclear [58–63]. Patients normally visit the hospital for a medical check-up during the day, which results in blood pressure monitoring. Isolated clinic blood pressure measurements from patients are not satisfactory to represent the daily blood pressure of the patients away from the medical environment over the last 50 years [64, 65]. Blood pressure measurement taken during daily activities by continuous ambulatory blood pressure monitoring will provide a more valid valuation of a patient's true blood pressure reading [66]. In addition, inconsistency in heart rate over 24 hours is an important indicator of the disease progression [67, 68]. Hence, a continuous monitoring medical system would be ideal for a patient to be aware of their health condition and to assist the doctor in prescribing treatment. A medical system to monitor and predict CVD is yet to be developed in the present-day context, as shown in Figure 2.6.

CVD is a term generally used to describe illness affecting the heart or blood vessels as well as other parts of the circulatory system. Coronary artery disease (CAD) is the common type of CVD that involves angina pectoris and myocardial infarction commonly known as heart attack [69]. Other types of

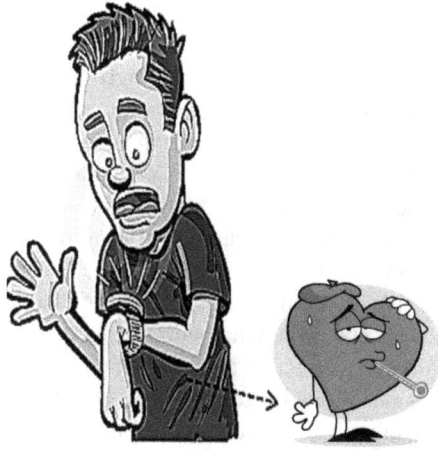

FIGURE 2.6 Medical system that would ensure continuous monitoring and prediction of cardiovascular disease.

CVDs include heart failure, stroke, rheumatic heart disease, venous thrombosis, peripheral artery disease, congenital heart disease, blood vessels disease, and heart valve disease [69, 70]. The underlying causes of these diseases include CAD, stroke, and diseases of the aorta and arteries, which are collectively known as atherosclerosis—a condition characterized by the narrowing of artery walls due to the deposition of fatty substances called atheroma [69]. The deposits cause the inner surface of the arteries to become irregular and narrow, hence disrupting the blood flow. Eventually, atheroma in the arteries can break away, causing the formation of a blood clot. When the blood clot blocks the artery that transports blood to the brain, the blood supply to the part of the brain is cut, thus causing stroke [59]. Similarly, when the blood clot occurs in the coronary artery, it can lead to a heart attack.

Several risk factors may contribute to an increased likelihood of developing CVDs, such as genetics, age, gender, ethnic background, smoking habits, high blood pressure, high blood cholesterol, obesity, and diabetes. While risk factors such as genetics, age, and gender are fixed in nature, the rest are volatile; thus, by making better choices, the outcome can be influenced. Inherited DNA sequence, which is a form of a fixed risk factor, increases the possibility of an offspring developing CVD by three times if the parent has a history of CVD [71]. Age, another fixed risk factor, is found to increase the CVD mortality rate parallel with it [71]. Besides that, mortality is also found to be higher by 2.3- to 2.7-fold for every decade of life for men and 2.9- to 3.7-fold for women in terms of gender [72]. The risk factor of gender also shows that men are more vulnerable to CVDs than premenopausal women [73] due to the estrogen hormone that is present in women, which improves the endothelial cell function and functions as a defense [74].

Meanwhile, modifiable risk factors such as high blood pressure, high blood cholesterol, and high lipid levels continue to play an extensive role in heart attacks and stroke. Lifestyle and behavioral changes such as mindful eating and implementing physical exercises into daily life are highly recommended. For instance, it is found that a diet rich in saturated fat leads to 31% of CHD and 11% stroke worldwide [75]. Thus, being more aware of the macro and micro values of daily food intake and altering it to suit respective body needs will significantly reduce the risk of getting CVDs. On top of that, it is also important for a person to be always updated on their current health status through regular medical check-ups for early detection and prevention.

Blood pressure is one of the biggest indicators of CVDs during a medical check-up. Blood pressure mirrors the contracting and relaxing of arterial walls that creates pressure waves, which is known as a pulse wave signal [76]. The pressure sensor is best at detecting arteriosclerosis, a condition of thickening and the hardening of blood vessels and deposition of plaque on the inner walls of the vessels that creates blocks and ultimately leads to cardiac arrest. Therefore, using the pressure sensor to detect and collect wrist pulse signals can assist in conducting further studies on better arteriosclerosis prediction [77, 78].

Besides arteriosclerosis, arrhythmia is another form of cardiac diseases that can be detected by using the same pulse wave signal. Arrhythmia is an abnormal electrical activity in the cardiovascular system. So, pulse wave signal can be used to detect this disease through the irregularity that will appear in the signal reflecting the increase and decrease of heart rate. In addition to that, the time variance that exists between continuous pulses exceeding the average level, incomplete waveforms, and merged waveform will also further help to detect arrhythmia by using pulse wave signal [79].

Medical
Technology

3

Constant and rapid technological advancement, especially in mobile and electronic healthcare, has significantly expanded the capabilities of physiological monitoring, such as the usage of wearable devices in recent times. A wearable device is a smart electronic device that is small enough to be worn on a human body and also able to incorporate powerful sensor technology for collecting and providing information about its surroundings. Wearable devices are currently used in healthcare services in the medical world, ranging from clinical-centric to patient-centric services, known as telemedicine. There are two types of telemedicine, namely live communication and store-and-forward. Live communication telemedicine functions by creating real-time communication between the doctor and the patient by using a wearable device that is equipped with high bandwidth and good data speed for timely data transmission. Meanwhile, store-and-forward telemedicine functions by collecting and storing the patient's medical data on their specific medical condition to be passed to the doctor for assessment upon request [80–83]. It has become easier for doctors to monitor a patient's body response constantly if the patient is using a wearable device [84–86]. Moreover, some intermediate level of local real-time classification is proposed by researchers, for example, the classification of heart rates by utilizing smartphones or personal digital assistants (PDAs) [87–90]. These methods have not yet given a total cardiovascular disease (CVD) diagnosis solution [91]. There are also telemedical functionalities through remote real-time monitoring system, where most of it uses (PDAs) to collect electrocardiography (ECG) where those signals are sent to a monitoring center for analysis and classification, subsequently denying the user the continuous outcome of their health [92–94].

Wearable devices are also useful to patients, as it gives the patient flexibility to carry out their daily routine while ensuring that their health is constantly monitored. When a patient performs various activities throughout the day, medical monitoring is widened as a bigger range of data can be obtained to provide better analysis for any conditions that may be present [95]. Patients who live further away from medical centers can benefit from using a wearable

DOI: 10.1201/9781003629832-3

device, as it allows monitoring of chronic CVDs such as heart attack by using a wireless monitoring system, reducing the patient's travelling frequency to hospitals [96]. Furthermore, a wearable device can also be made an integral part of routine care for acute or chronic diseases, as it will provide information to both the hospital and the patient, raising the awareness level of both parties on the patient's health condition [83]. Several wireless and sensor technologies have been developed, such as finger-ring sensors [97], smartwatches [98], and mobile applications [99, 100], to help patients understand and control their heart conditions in their daily lives. Studies show that patients who are more aware of their health condition tend to give higher importance to bettering their lifestyle and habits [101, 102].

The common way of monitoring health conditions is to monitor a person's blood pressure. In today's technological era, the wearable device can monitor a person's blood pressure. This wearable device is placed at the user's wrist where the radial artery is located. There are three types of sensors that are used universally to measure radial blood pressure waveform, which are pressure sensor such as applanation tonometry, photoelectric sensor such as plethysmography, and ultrasonic sensors such as Doppler. Table 3.1 shows the currently available medical technologies and their type of sensors. Table 3.2 shows the accuracy, sensitivity, and specificity of the three types of sensors, which are pressure, photoelectric, and ultrasound sensor.

After comparing these three electronic sensors through Table 3.2, it can be concluded that the pressure sensor may best suit the need to develop the medical device for continuous monitoring. The pressure sensor has the best accuracy, sensitivity, and specificity to detect radial pulse waves compared to the photoelectric and ultrasonic sensors. Pressure sensor also echoes the way a traditional diagnosis is done to a certain extent, besides generating pulse wave signals with less noise as compared to the photoelectric sensor and ultrasonic sensor.

3.1 PRESSURE SENSOR

The pressure sensor is a type of sensor that is used to determine the transmural pressure at the radial blood vessel to obtain the wrist pulse signal [135, 136]. Figure 3.1 shows the radial pulse wave signal that was formed using pressure sensors. Figure 3.2 shows the parameters that can be read through a pressure sensor.

There are a lot of researchers working on pressure sensor. For example, Sharmila et al. [136] have done research on diagnosing diseases through radial pulse wave signals using a pressure sensor. The research objective was to obtain a radial pulse wave signal from the wrist and relate it to the Indian traditional

TABLE 3.1 Current available medical technologies for measuring central blood pressure

MEDICAL TECHNOLOGY	TYPE OF CARE	SITE OF RECORD	TYPE OF SENSOR	ESTIMATION METHOD	PRESSURE CALIBRATION	INVASIVE VALIDATION	FDA APPROVAL
ABPM 7100Welch Allyn, Inc (acquired by Hillrom)	Ambulatory care	Brachial artery	Brachial cuff pulse volume plethysmography	Generalize transfer function	Brachial cuff SBP/DBP	No	No
ARCsolver + VaSeraVS-1500Austrian Institute of Technology, Austria	Nonambulatory care	Brachial artery	Brachial cuff pulse volume plethysmography	Generalize transfer function	Brachial cuff SBP/DBP	Yes [103]	Yes
Arteriograph 24 h, TensioMED Ltd., Hungary	Ambulatory care	Brachial artery	Suprasystolic brachial cuff plethysmography	SBP2 + regression	Brachial cuff MAP/DBP	Yes [104, 105]	No
Arteriograph TensioMed Ltd., Hungary	Nonambulatory care	Brachial artery	Suprasystolic brachial cuff plethysmography	SBP2 + regression	Brachial cuff MAP/DBP	Yes	No
BP + Uscom Ltd., Australia (acquire Pulsecor Ltd., Cardioscope II)	Nonambulatory care	Brachial artery	Suprasystolic brachial cuff plethysmography	Physical model Brachial suprasystolic waveform	Brachial cuff SBP/DBP	Yes [106]	No

(continued)

TABLE 3.1 (Continued)

MEDICAL TECHNOLOGY	TYPE OF CARE	SITE OF RECORD	TYPE OF SENSOR	ESTIMATION METHOD	PRESSURE CALIBRATION	INVASIVE VALIDATION	FDA APPROVAL
BPLab Petr Telegin, Russia	Nonambulatory care	Brachial artery	Brachial cuff pulse volume plethysmography	Generalize transfer function	Brachial cuff SBP/DBP	Yes [107]	Yes
BPro + A-Pulse, HealthSTATS, Singapore (acquired by Hillrom)	Ambulatory care	Radial artery	Applanation tonometry Single, fixed (watch type)	N-point moving average	Brachial cuff SBP/DBP	Yes [108–110]	Yes
cBP301Centron Diagnostics, UK (acquired by SunTech Medical)	Nonambulatory care	Brachial artery	Brachial cuff plethysmography	GTF	Brachial cuff SBP/DBP	Yes [111]	Yes
Complior Alam Medical, France	Nonambulatory care	Carotid artery	Applanation tonometry, Single, fixed	Simple substitution	Brachial cuff MAP/DBP	Yes [112]	No
DynaPulse Pulse Metric Inc, USA	Nonambulatory care	Brachial artery	Suprasystolic brachial cuff plethysmography	Physical model	Brachial cuff SBP/DBP	Yes [113]	Yes
GaonHanbyul Meditech, Korea	Non-Ambulatory care	Radial artery	Applanation tonometry Single, fixed	Generalize Transfer Function	Brachial cuff SBP/DBP	Yes [114]	Yes

Device	Care	Artery	Method	Calibration	Reference		
HEM-9000AI Omron Healthcare, Japan	Non-Ambulatory care	Radial artery	Applanation tonometry Arrayed [115], fixed	SBP2 + regression	Brachial cuff SBP/DBP	Yes [116–119]	No
Mobil-O-Graph NGI.EM GmbH, Germany	Ambulatory care	Brachial artery	Brachial cuff pulse volume plethysmography	Generalize Transfer Function	Brachial cuff SBP/DBP	Yes [120]	Yes
Mobil-O-GraphI.EM GmbH, Germany Brachialartery	Nonambulatory care	Brachial artery	Brachial cuff pulse volume plethysmography	Generalize Transfer Function	Brachial cuff SBP/DBP	Yes [120]	Yes
NIHem Cardiovascular Engineering Inc, USA	NonAmbulatory care	Carotid artery	Applanation tonometry, Single, manual	Simple substitution	Brachial cuff MAP/DBP	Yes [121]	No
Oscar 2 with SphygmoCor SunTech Medical, USABrachial	Nonambulatory care	Brachial artery	Subdiastolic brachial cuff plethysmography	Generalize Transfer Function	Brachial cuff SBP/DBP	Yes	Yes
Oscar 2 with SphygmoCor, SunTech Medical	Ambulatory care	Brachial artery	Subdiastolic brachial cuff plethysmography	Generalize Transfer Function	Brachial cuff SBP/DBP	Yes [122]	Yes
PulsePen DiaTecne srl., Italy	Nonambulatory care	Carotid artery	Applanation tonometry Single, manual	Simple substitution	Brachial cuff MAP/DBP	Yes [123]	No

(continued)

TABLE 3.1 (Continued)

MEDICAL TECHNOLOGY	TYPE OF CARE	SITE OF RECORD	TYPE OF SENSOR	ESTIMATION METHOD	PRESSURE CALIBRATION	INVASIVE VALIDATION	FDA APPROVAL
SphygmoCor XCELAtCor Medical, Australia	Nonambulatory care	Brachial artery	Subdiastolic brachial cuff plethysmography	Generalize transfer function	Brachial cuff SBP/DBP	Yes [124]	Yes
Sphygmo CorCVMS, AtCor Medical, Australia	Nonambulatory care	Radial artery	Applanation tonometry Single, manual	Generalize transfer function	Brachial cuff SBP/DBP	Yes [108, 119, 120, 125130]	Yes
Vicorder Skidmore Medical Ltd., UK	Nonambulatory care	Brachial artery	Brachial cuff pulse volume plethysmography	Generalize transfer function	Brachial cuff MAP/DBP	Yes [127, 131]	Yes
WatchBP Microlife Corp, Taiwan	Nonambulatory care	Brachial artery	Brachial cuff pulse volume plethysmography	(SBP2, DBP, As, Ad) + regression	Brachial cuff SBP/DBP	Yes [132, 133]	Yes
WatchBP O3, Microlife AG, Widnau, Switzerland	Ambulatory care	Brachial artery	Brachial cuff pulse volume plethysmography	(SBP2, DBP, As, Ad) + regression	Brachial cuff SBP/DBP	Yes [134]	Yes

TABLE 3.2   Diagnosis performance of the three types of sensor

	ACCURACY (%)	SENSITIVITY (%)	SPECIFICITY (%)
Pressure	86.4	87.6	85.2
Photoelectric	79.3	83.1	75.8
Ultrasonic	83.7	85.4	82.1
Combination of three types of signals	89.7	91.0	88.4

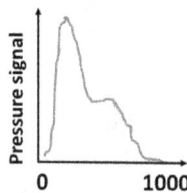

FIGURE 3.1   Radial pulse wave obtained from pressure sensor.

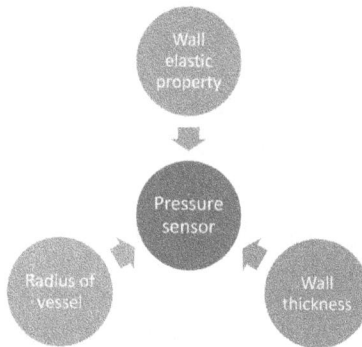

FIGURE 3.2   Parameters obtained by pressure sensor.

method of diagnosis. The Indian traditional method takes the pulse from the wrist by using three fingertips. The three energies that significantly influence the pulse rhythms that can be detected using the fingertips are called kapha, pitta, and vata. Therefore, three pressure transducers were attached at the wrist to obtain the three pulses. The first sensor that was used was '1 PS1' pressure sensor from 'Sensym Products'. This was a failure as it was unable to capture the intricacies of the pulse. Therefore, 'Millivolt Output Medium Pressure Sensor' form Mouser Electronics, Inc was used. There is a tiny diaphragm at the center that has a '0–4 inches H2O' pressure range. The data were captured with a sampling rate of 500 Hz by 16-bit multifunction data acquisition card NI USB-6210 which interlinks to collect data from the pressure sensor. Lab view was used as the data acquisition software to control the digitization. The research had two phases [136].

Suket et al. had used a pressure sensor to obtain a radial pulse wave signal. The work was mainly about wrist pulse acquisition and recording system. The pressure sensor that was used for this project was MPXM2053D piezo-resistive pressure sensor [137]. Along the line, ARM Cortex M4 architecture was used for digitization of signals and fed into the LCD for real-time monitoring. The signals were recorded onto a micro-SD memory card for offline processing and analysis. The purpose of the project was to have a better understanding of the wrist pulse wave signal and support the ayurvedic practitioner to detect pulse wave signals [138].

Research about flexible polymer transistors with high-pressure sensitivity for application in electronic skin and health monitoring was done by Gregor Schwartz, et al. The research was aimed towards developing a pressure sensor by using polydimethylsiloxane (PDMS) material. PDMS materials are from a group of polymeric organosilicon compounds, which are also known as silicones. The sensor was fabricated in the form of pyramids of 3 mm height, 6 mm base length, and 8.85 mm spacing. The sensor showed that it had a response time of less than 10 ms due to the effect of the microstructured PDMS dielectric upon pressure release [139].

Choon Meng Ting and Ngak Hwee Chua invented Bpro watch which functions as a radial pulse wave acquisition device. This device can be used on either the right or left wrist to obtain the radial pulse wave signal. The watch measures in 10-second intervals to obtain a block of the radial pulse wave signal. It can be connected through Bluetooth to ease data transfer and weighs only around 60 g. However, it has a memory to save only 96 blocks of radial pulse wave signals. The watch monitors systolic and diastolic blood pressure, heart rate, central aortic systolic pressure, and 24-hour blood pressure patterns. The watch currently can only diagnose hypertensive patients [140, 141].

3.2 PHOTOELECTRIC SENSOR

The photoelectric sensor, on the other hand, is used to measure the blood volume at the radial blood vessel by transmitting light and receiving the signal by the reflected light, which is in proportion with the volume of the vessel. Figure 3.3 shows the radial pulse wave signal that was formed using photoelectric sensors. Figure 3.4 shows the parameters that can be read through a photoelectric sensor.

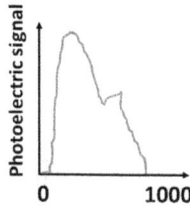

FIGURE 3.3 Radial pulse wave obtained from photoelectric sensor.

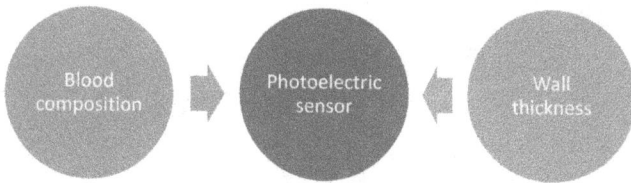

FIGURE 3.4 Parameters obtained by photoelectric sensor.

Photoelectric sensors have various designs, but all of it provides similar results where they measure the change in blood volume [142]. The change in blood volume is measured by the LEDs emitting light and using the photodiode to measure the intensity of the nonabsorbed light reflected from tissue [143]. Red and green are the most common LED colors used in most studies, but there are some studies showing yellow LED being used [144]. The LED light which has longer wavelengths will be able to penetrate more deeply into the tissue such as infrared light. It can penetrate deeper compared to the green light LED [145]. The infrared light which has longer wavelength does have its disadvantage that it is more prone to motion artifacts. Motion artifact is a patient-based artifact that occurs with voluntary or involuntary patient movement during data acquisition. Hence, a green light LED which has a shorter wavelength would be a better option in certain applications [145]. To avoid motion artifact, wearable devices nowadays are equipped with accelerometers to record the movements [144] especially during physical activity.

3.3 ULTRASONIC SENSOR

The ultrasonic sensor, which works similarly to the photoelectric sensor, uses sound waves rather than light to measure the blood velocity in the vessel [77, 135]. Figure 3.5 shows the radial pulse wave signal that was formed using

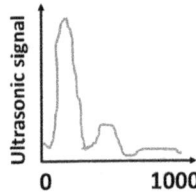

FIGURE 3.5 Radial pulse wave obtained from ultrasonic sensor.

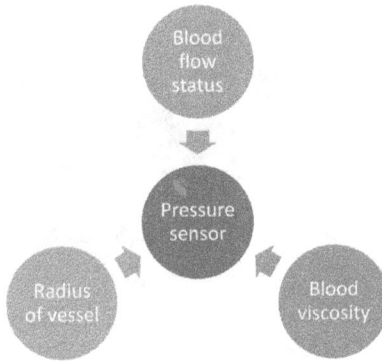

FIGURE 3.6 Parameters obtained by ultrasonic sensor.

ultrasonic sensors. Figure 3.6 shows the parameters that can be measured through an ultrasonic sensor. The ultrasonic waves can effectively penetrate human tissues up to a depth of 4 cm, which allows better sensing range in today's technology [146]. Moreover, the main frequency is less than 12 Hz [147] for blood pressure waveforms, which is lower than the 10 MHz frequency range of a typical ultrasonic device. An ultrasonic device can safeguard a conformal close contact with the curved skin surface when acquiring a blood pressure waveform, which reduces the difficulty or instability compared to the other methods [146]. The ultrasonic sensor is similar to the cardiac ultrasound process, where it uses high-frequency sound wave. In Doppler ultrasound, it uses an electrical signal source [148] to produce the ultrasonic wave transmitted through the human body. The Doppler effect occurs when there is a change in frequency. This happens when the red blood cells move into the bloodstream where the change in time from one position to another is related to the frequency shift, which shows a positive or negative change depending on the direction of the blood flow. Hence, with an ultrasonic sensor, the direction of blood flow can be determined.

Diagnosing Cardiovascular Diseases

4

Methods and procedures of diagnosing cardiovascular diseases (CVDs) can be divided into two main categories, which are invasive methods and noninvasive methods. The invasive methods comprise the use of technological equipment that punchers the human body, whereas the noninvasive method does not have or requires minimal contact with the human body. The invasive methods are conducted by experts in the medical field to ensure the safety of the patients. Modern diagnosis methods implement both invasive and noninvasive methods to diagnose CVDs, whereas traditional diagnosis methods focus on diagnosing CVDs by noninvasive methods.

4.1 TRADITIONAL DIAGNOSIS METHOD

The two most common traditional methods are traditional Chinese medicine (TCM) and ayurveda (ancient Indian medicine). TCM's constitutional taxonomy system originates from China, which is associated with the weather and elemental classification [149, 150]. The ideas (Yin, Yang, and Qi) in TCM are convoluted, as a result of most of the principles of TCM being influenced by Chinese philosophy [150, 151]. The principles of Yin and Yang are the main perception of TCM. These principles are the two opposite states of the body that are complementary, dependent, and interchangeable with one another [152, 153]. Within the process of diagnosis and treatment, these principles have already been internalized into the medical theory supported by TCM, which could be a construct of scientific theory [153]. These principles of the body are maintained in a balanced state. Attacks by exogenous pathogens, debility, emotional stress, or exhaustion may disturb the balance between the principles and

DOI: 10.1201/9781003629832-4

may lead to diseases. TCM syndrome (also known as Zheng) could be a state that may be assessed by review, listening, olfaction, interrogation, and palpation [153]. The information on 'palpation' is the assessment of the pulse, which is used in traditional and modern practice. The pulse is commonly obtained at the radial artery located at the wrist for the traditional method to be analyzed for diagnostic purpose. This method is known as Chinese pulse diagnosis (CPD). CPD otherwise called Shen–Hammer pulse diagnosing is the system of pulse diagnosis used by Dr John H. F. Shen, OMD, and documented in a present-day approach by Dr Leon Hammer, MD, within the book Chinese Pulse diagnosing [154, 155]. This pulse system is based on an exceedingly long history of Chinese medical data that existed in China before the Communist Revolution [155–157]. The secrets prized by the historic family lineages were closely guarded for reasons of success and survival. Those without direct inheritance of the oral tradition had very little or no access to the knowledge. Exceptional circumstances occurring in recent history have allowed folks outside the lineage access to the current knowledge of CPD [99].

On the other hand, ayurvedic medication is the ancient medical system of India that relies on Tridoshic theory. The three doshas are vata, pitta, and kapha [158]. The three doshas are forces that contain completely different proportions of the five parts of air, fire, earth, ether, and water [159, 160]. The psychobiological tendencies in ayurveda are termed Prakruti and refer to the inherent balance of a singular combination of mental and physical qualities that show up as foreseeable patterns within the mind–body system of a person [159, 160]. This ideal constitutional balance of a person is set at birth and grossly correlates with the individual's patterns of the organic phenomenon [161, 162]. Ayurvedic theories read that the psychobiological tendencies of every Prakruti possess innate vulnerabilities to concern and unhealthiness [159–163]. It is understood that once the psychobiological tendencies of the fundamental constitution are out of balance, unhealthiness is next to be reckoned [159, 162].

These traditional medicines diagnose CVDs by studying a patient's wrist pulse signal. To do so, pulses are felt by placing three fingers namely the index, middle, and ring finger on the radial artery, which is located on the right forearm, 2 cm up from the wrist [164]. This is visualized in Figure 4.1 for a traditional method of diagnosis. The right wrist is used for the male and the left wrist is used for a female to check the pulse wave [165]. A healthy human would have three pulse amplitudes in the ratio of 4:2:1, respectively, but this could change depending on the seasonal variation and other factors such as time of day, temperature, and humidity of the skin. Some of these pulse characteristics are summarized in Figure 4.1.

Unlike modern medicine methodology where practitioners' take into consideration only the pulse rate, traditional medicine practitioners' look into the energies that are circulating in a human's body, namely the kapha, pitta, and vata energy that influences the rhythm of the pulse as well. Analyzing these

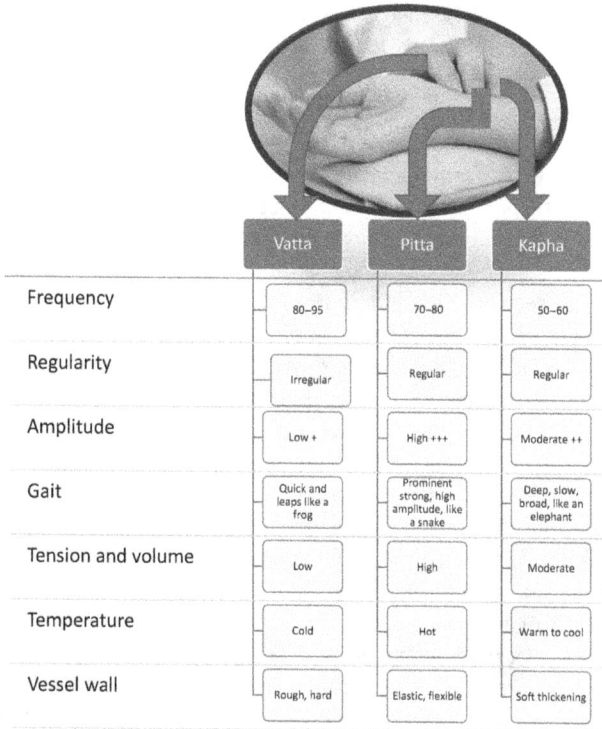

	Vatta	Pitta	Kapha
Frequency	80–95	70–80	50–60
Regularity	Irregular	Regular	Regular
Amplitude	Low +	High +++	Moderate ++
Gait	Quick and leaps like a frog	Prominent strong, high amplitude, like a snake	Deep, slow, broad, like an elephant
Tension and volume	Low	High	Moderate
Temperature	Cold	Hot	Warm to cool
Vessel wall	Rough, hard	Elastic, flexible	Soft thickening

FIGURE 4.1   The process of pulse diagnosis and the characteristics of pulses.

pulse patterns through their rhythm is the key to disease identification in traditional medicine [166]. In fact, using this traditional method of diagnosis, a traditional practitioner can identify up to 350 different diseases. However, obtaining a patient's wrist pulse signal by this technique is very subjective due to different perspectives of the individual practitioners. Besides, this method also takes years of practice as a practitioner to develop skills to sense the wrist pulse signal by the three fingertips beforehand and to use the sense of familiarity to match the patient's signal to a diseased signal that he may have come across before to conclude the CVD of the patient [138, 167–169].

4.2 MODERN DIAGNOSIS METHOD

Modern diagnosis methods detect the heart's abnormalities by diagnosis using various types of clinical testing. The three most common modern methods are electrocardiogram (ECG), medical imaging, and blood pressure (BP). The ECG is a method that records the electrical activity of the heart. This ECG readings are acquired using an electrode at specific points of the body such as the chest, wrist, and ankles where there are six electrodes placed in the chest and four placed in the limb or periphery, where one of the electrodes is 'neutral'. Hence, ten wires are connected from the ECG machine to the human body, which registers the signals and then produces an output showing the electrical activity of the heart. Figure 4.2 shows the placement of ECG electrodes, while Figure 4.3 shows the output ECG signal obtained by the electrodes.

As can be seen in Figure 4.3, P wave represents atrial depolarization, QRS segment represents ventricular depolarization, Q wave represents the first downward wave of the QRS complex where the Q wave is normally absent, R wave represents the initial positive deflection, S wave represents the negative deflection following the R wave, and the T wave represents ventricular repolarization. This information is about each phases of the heart beat. The ECG signal provides a valuable information of the heart because its electrical wave indicates the contraction of each muscles in the heart, which reciprocates with the rhythm of the heartbeat. Therefore, irregularities in heart rate and rhythm that result from the heart being overworked, and more importantly, the progression of heart attacks can be detected by using ECG [170, 171]. A Holter monitor or other ambulatory ECG would be more suitable for certain cases as the tests are able to record the electrical activity of the heart during daily activities whereas the ECG records the heart activity at only one point in time. A Holter monitor in the form of a small portable battery-powered ECG machine is able to record heartbeats over a period of 24–48 hours, or longer, during normal activities. This portable device is useful for monitoring slow, fast, or irregular heartbeat, abnormal heart rhythms and cardiac symptoms, effect of medication, pacemaker function, and so on [170–173]. In addition, medical imaging is another modern medicine technique to identify CVD. There are many types of medical imaging methods used for diagnostic purposes based on the visual information obtained from specific parts of the body. Common medical imaging procedures used for CVD patients include the echocardiogram, X-ray, CT scan, and MRI scan. The echocardiogram otherwise known as cardiac ultrasound uses high frequency ultrasound waves for imaging. The echocardiogram has a transducer probe, which is placed over the chest. This transducer produces sound waves that bounce off the heart, which results in the echo reflections back to the probe. These reflected signals then produce an output image that can be viewed on a video monitor. The echocardiogram allows the medical specialists to determine the size, shape, thickness, and movement of heart walls, movement, and pumping strength of the heart. Additionally, the echocardiogram can be used to determine the condition of the heart valves if there is leaking backwards (regurgitation), valves are too

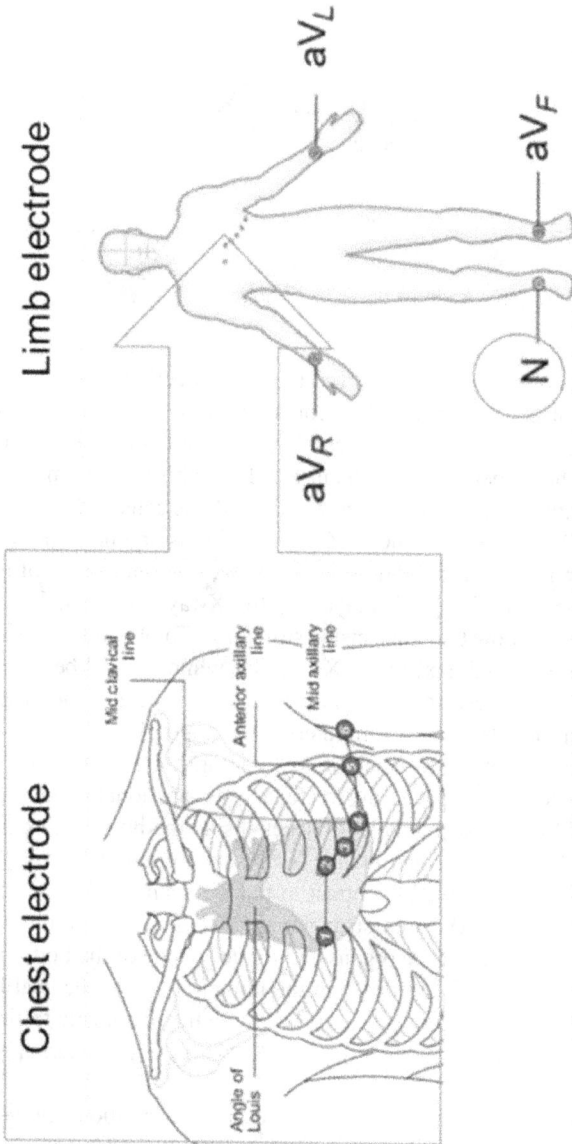

Limb electrode

aV$_L$

aV$_R$

aV$_F$

N

Chest electrode

Mid clavical line

Anterior axillary line

Mid axillary line

Angle of Louis

FIGURE 4.2 Placement of ECG electrodes.

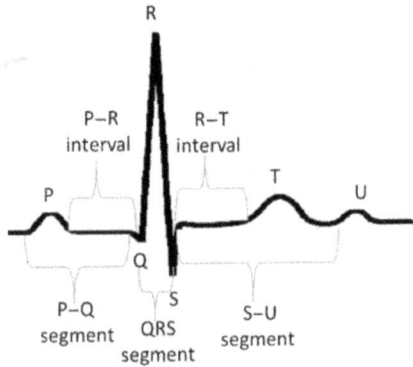

FIGURE 4.3   Example section of an ECG signal.

narrow (stenosis), or the presence of a tumor or infectious growth around the valves. Medical experts utilize the echocardiogram to investigate problems with the pericardium, large blood vessels, blood clots in the heart chambers, and abnormal holes between the chambers. The echocardiogram is known to be safe for testing as there are no known side effects caused by the procedure up to date [174–176]. Furthermore, X-ray imaging is another type of medical imaging which is used to determine the location, size, and shape of the heart, lungs, and blood. The image displayed by the X-ray shows the bones of the chest but does not show the other inside structures. To obtain the X-ray image, the patient is positioned next to the X-ray film while a small beam of X-rays passes through the chest and makes an image on special photographic film [177, 178]. On the other hand, computerized tomography (CT) scan is a type of medical imaging where a series of X-ray images are taken from different angles and use computer processing to create cross-sectional images, or slices, of the bones, blood vessels, and soft tissues inside the body. CT scan images provide more detailed information than X-rays by merging the cross-sectional images of the X-rays [179]. In contrast to the CT scan and X-rays, magnetic resonance imaging (MRI) uses strong magnetic fields and radio waves to produce detailed images of the organs and tissues inside of the body. The MRI is taken with the patient lying down in the tunnel [180]. In medical imaging, the different types of imaging play a role to suite the diagnostic testing of the relevant CVD to help the medical experts to visualize the internal image of the organ.

The measurement of BP is generally presented as a ratio of two numbers. An example of a healthy BP measurement is 120/80 mmHg [181]. The first or the larger number represents the systolic BP in the arteries during contraction of the heart muscles, whereas the second number or the smaller number indicates the pressure in the arteries during the resting period in between the heartbeats when the heart relaxes and refills with blood. BP generally represents the arterial BP, which is the pressure between the aorta and its branches. Pulse pressure is the difference between the systolic and diastolic BP. Noninvasively, the BP is commonly measured using a sphygmomanometer in a clinical setting [182]. Cardiac output, blood volume, peripheral resistance, and viscosity are the four key factors that influence BP. When these four key factors increase, the BP will increase respectively. A healthy condition of the cardiovascular system can be determined by the BP reading, where if the readings obtained are higher than the average BP in normal conditions, it will indicate aortic stiffness due to atherosclerosis. In this condition, the patient will most likely develop hypertension, which will result in an increase in heart disease and stroke. On the other hand, low BP may indicate that the heart or the valve is functioning poorly.

Currently in modern diagnosis, patients showing distinctive indications can be exposed to extra tests, different types of imaging [183, 184] and invasive techniques such as angiogram are done for a more conclusive diagnosis, despite the fact that they can convey critical dangers that must be deliberately gauged [185]. This invasive method where a part of the body is catheterized, either by puncture or incision, is the current diagnosis for CVD. This medical procedure is painful as well as time-consuming for patients with CVD or suspected of CVD. Current diagnostic tools for CVDs also have drawbacks, as most of the technology is not portable, consumes space, and needs a doctor's consultation. In general, there is a solid requirement for reliable diagnostics and a safe, nonobtrusive medical system that can be utilized as an early detection tool to give precise information about CVD development over time. This would ease people with CVD who are not able to identify their illness until the symptoms show an obvious sign, usually at the critical stage, which results in a high risk of mortality. On the other hand, patients with diagnosed CVDs are also concerned with their health status, but frequent visits to the hospital to monitor their health are rather inconvenient. Therefore, the development of a medical system to monitor and predict CVD will lay a foundation to resolve the above-mentioned problems owing to CVD and promote advances in several biomedical devices for continuous monitoring and early detection of CVD.

Cardiovascular Disease Detection and AI Integration

5

Cardiovascular disease (CVD) detection or risk indication has been practiced by hospitals, where the common approach of noninvasive indication of hypertension relating to cardiovascular risk for further investigation is done by attaining the central aortic blood pressure's systolic and diastolic reading. This is done by using the brachial oscillometer in the hospital. With today's development of medical wearable devices, the central aortic blood pressure waveform can be estimated from the peripheral artery, which would allow continuous monitoring. Furthermore, CVD can be indicated by using various types of risk indication scores, and this risk indication score can be incorporated with artificial intelligence (AI).

5.1 CENTRAL AORTIC BLOOD PRESSURE WAVEFORM FOR DETECTION OF CVD

In hospital practice, the blood pressure is measured using the brachial oscillometer [186–189] where the reading of the brachial artery is considered the same as the central aortic pressure (CAP) by clinicians [124]. Even though the brachial artery is close to the aorta artery, the brachial blood pressure waveform reading is not the same as the CAP waveform due to the wave reflection, systolic blood pressure, diastolic blood pressure, pulse pressure, and mean artery pressure. It is known that the blood pressure at the aorta and peripheral artery such as the brachial artery differs for the pulse pressure, diastolic blood pressure, and mean artery pressure. Where the pulse pressure increases from

DOI: 10.1201/9781003629832-5

the aorta to the peripheral artery while the mean artery pressure and diastolic blood pressure decrease by 1–2 mmHg from the aorta to the peripheral arteries [190–192]. CAP waveforms have the factors of cardiac loading and perfusion, which are important for cardiovascular function [125]. Information about this waveform is often crucial for precise monitoring and diagnosis of CVDs [125]. Recent research evidence has shown that cardiovascular outcomes can be strongly related to the CAP [64, 193–202]. For instance, Agabiti-Rosei et al. has conducted research showing that the central pressure has a closer correlation with surrogate measures of CVD [64]. Furthermore, conduit artery function evaluation (CAFE) has studied the differential effects of interventions on central and peripheral pressure [203] and has shown that CAP provides a superior measure of hemodynamic load on the heart and central organs. CAP is commonly used to determine hypertension. Besides that, CAP has given insights into the prevention, diagnosis, and treatment of CVDs, including coronary artery disease, stroke, myocardial infarction, and heart failure [124]. Measurement of CAP is usually conducted invasively, which is not ideal for continuous monitoring or to be used as a screening tool. In today's technological world, there are commercialized wearable devices that estimates the CAP noninvasively from the peripheral artery. These wearable devices are strapped at the user's wrist to acquire the radial blood pressure waveform and estimate the CAP. Current wearable devices utilize the radial blood pressure waveform as it would be comfortable to the user, and also calibration of systolic and diastolic blood pressure using cuff-sphygmomanometric is more suitable for applying the tonometry technique at the upper limb site such as radial artery compared to another peripheral artery such as carotid artery due to the pulse pressure amplification [204]. In addition, the bony structure (radius) underlying the radial artery gives an advantage compared to other peripheral arteries, where it ensures an easy and optimal applanation tonometry [204]. However, radial blood pressure waveforms must be mathematically transformed in order to attain the central aortic blood pressure waveform [204].

5.1.1 Generalized Transfer Function

The common way of converting a radial pulse wave signal to the aortic wave signal is by using "generalized transfer functions" (GTF) [125, 205–211]. GTF in the time or frequency domain is used to obtain the central aortic waveform from the radial waveform by relating the aortic hemodynamic indices [125, 205, 206]. This technique assumes the relationship between the radial blood pressure waveform, and the aortic blood pressure waveform is kept the same for a set of subjects with similar physiological and pathological characteristics [124]. However, errors occur when applying a GTF generated from one specific group of patients to another group with different ages undergoing different treatment [207, 208]. The error caused by GTF is very dependent on the heart rate and blood pressure level. Hence, this should be taken into consideration when the GTF is applied to a set of subjects with different hemodynamic conditions [212]. SphygmoCorCVMS, AtCor Medical, Australia [108, 119, 120] was the first device accepted by the US Food and Drug Administration (FDA) that utilized GTF to estimate the central aortic blood pressure waveform. This commercial device calculates the GTF by using multiple central and peripheral blood pressure waveforms, which undergo a Fourier analysis. This device obtains the peripheral pressure waveform from the user, which is converted to the frequency domain and multiplied with the calculated GTF. The result of this is then converted back to the time domain to obtain the estimated central aortic blood pressure waveform [120, 126, 130, 206, 213, 214]. The research conducted on 30 patients by Cloud et al. [215] has shown that the GTF method by SphygmoCor for estimating the central aortic blood pressure waveform underestimates the systolic pressure and overestimates the diastolic pressure of the CAP by 13.3 and 11.5 mmHg, respectively. Since the SphygmoCor method underestimates the systolic blood pressure, it may not be suited to determine patients for hypertension because it is known that systolic blood pressure is a better predictor of hypertension risk [216] which relates to cardiac disease.

5.1.2 N-Point Moving Average

A simpler method of accessing the central aortic blood pressure waveform compared to the GTF is the N-point moving average (NPMA). The NPMA is a first-order low-pass filter where it removes all the high-frequency-related pulse wave features as it travels from the central aorta to the periphery [124]. The high-frequency features that are removed by NPMA are related to the wave reflections, and the NPMA provides the central aortic systolic blood pressure reading instead of the aortic blood pressure waveform [124]. The N-point moving average (NPMA) with a denominator of one-quarter of the tonometer sampling frequency accurately defines the CAP when applied to noninvasively acquired radial signals from the patient [109], which is utilized by BPro+A-Pulse, HealthSTATS [108–110]. This method is also a generalized method where it will contribute error for subject variability.

5.1.3 Adaptive Transfer Function

An adaptive transfer function (ATF) was created by Gao et al to address the limitation of GTF's population averages, where the GTF is not able to adapt to the variations in the ratio of radial to aortic pulse pressure (pulse pressure (PP) amplification) [217]. There are several ATF methods proposed to tune the GTF to obtain a more reliable CAP [218, 219]. The simple ATF for deriving the central blood pressure waveform from a radial blood pressure waveform, which was developed by Gao et al. was able to give greater accuracy than GTF in the low pulse pressure amplification subjects while showing a similar accuracy with high pulse pressure amplification subjects [217]. This ATF is a model-based transfer function where it takes into consideration the wave travel time and wave reflection coefficient parameters of a physiologic model of arterial wave transmission and reflection [217]. From the research by Gao et al, it is known that the ATF is not able to improve the estimation of the augmentation index and ejection interval of the central blood pressure waveform. This is due to the physiological model being developed by two parameters, which is too simple to adapt to the detailed features of the central blood pressure waveform [217].

5.1.4 Second Systolic Pressure of Periphery

The attained radial or brachial blood pressure waveform can directly estimate the systolic blood pressure reading of the central aortic blood pressure waveform by analyzing the second systolic pressure of the periphery (radial or brachial). The reflected wave peak of the radial or brachial blood pressure waveform approximates the systolic pressure of the aortic blood pressure waveform because the pressure gradient in the blood flow from the central aortic to the peripheral is relatively small during late systole where the late systolic shoulder represents the dominant peak in most adults in their midlife [116, 220]. On the other hand, systolic blood pressure of the central aortic blood pressure waveform for older adults [126] can be calculated using a regression equation where the second systolic pressure of the periphery will act as an independent variable [117, 221]. The technique of utilizing the second systolic pressure of the periphery to directly estimate the systolic blood pressure reading of the central aortic blood pressure waveform is used by the commercial device HEM-9000AI Omron Healthcare, Japan [116–119]. The limitation of this technique is that it will not work when the second peak of the periphery disappears, which normally occurs in old patients and patients with hypertension or arterial stiffness [124]. In addition, this technique depends on the morphology of the peripheral waveform (radial or brachial blood pressure waveform) to estimate the CAP. Hence, the systolic blood pressure of the central aortic would be inaccurate for younger individuals with nonaugmented peak systolic pressure [118].

5.1.5 Summary on Estimation of Central Aortic Blood Pressure Waveform

From the above findings, it is known that the majority of the wearable ambulatory devices are utilizing a GTF to estimate the central aortic blood pressure waveform such as Mobil-O-Graph NGI.EM GmbH, Germany [120], Oscar 2 with SphygmoCor, SunTech Medical [122], and ABPM 7100Welch Allyn, Inc. There are wearable ambulatory devices that are utilizing the second systolic pressure of the periphery with regression to estimate the systolic blood pressure reading such as Arteriograph 24 h, TensioMED Ltd., Hungary [104, 105], and WatchBP O3, Microlife AG, Widnau, Switzerland [134]. Besides that, there is the BPro + A-Pulse, HealthSTATS, Singapore [108–110] which utilizes the N-NPMA to estimate the central aortic blood pressure waveform. The research conducted on 30 patients by Cloud et al. [215] has shown that the GTF method by SphygmoCor for estimating the central aortic blood pressure waveform underestimates the systolic pressure, and it may not be suited to determine patients for hypertension because it is known that systolic blood pressure is a better predictor of hypertension risk [216]. Moreover, the ambulatory devices that utilize second systolic pressure of the periphery to estimate the central aortic blood pressure waveform will not work when the second peak of the periphery disappears, which normally occurs in old patients and patients with hypertension or arterial stiffness [124]. The NPMA technique utilized by the Bpro watch provides the central aortic systolic blood pressure reading instead of the aortic blood pressure waveform [124]. In addition, all the current commercialized ambulatory devices utilize these techniques using software in the central processing unit (CPU) to convert the radial to aortic blood pressure waveform, where the device is acquiring the radial blood pressure signal and transmitting the data to the computer to process the conversion of the radial blood pressure waveform to the aortic blood pressure waveform for analysis of the signal and indication of hypertension. For example, the BPro wearable watch, which is an ambulatory device, acquires the radial blood pressure waveform and transfers the acquired data via Bluetooth or cable to the computer, where the + A-Pulse Health STATS software with NPMA converts the acquired signal to an estimated aortic blood pressure waveform for analysis. Hence, there is a need to identify a current method or develop a novel method with low computational intensity that is able to give a close estimate of the actual aortic blood pressure waveform with a close prediction of the systolic pressure that can be embedded in the user's watch (microcontroller) to ensure continuous conversion of central aortic blood pressure waveform. Then, the estimated central aortic blood pressure waveform can be directly analyzed to indicate the risk to the user without the need to transmit data to a computer or any cloud platforms. This will ensure that the user is always aware of their health even if there isn't any Wifi, Bluetooth, or wireless communication to a computer or cloud platforms for processing and analysis.

5.2 RISK INDICATION FOR CVD

CVD risk indication scores were initially conducted in the Framingham study [222] which was used to predict an individual's cardiovascular risk by using variables such as age, gender, cholesterol, smoking habit, blood pressure levels, etc. This Framingham technique in indicating risk of CVDs had certain methodological drawbacks when it was applied to different populations around the world (Seven Countries Study dataset) such as overestimates risk in young people and overpredicting absolute risk in low-risk European populations, which was identified by Menotti et al. [223] in the early 2000s. To address the drawbacks when applying risk indication to different population sizes and types, the European Society of Cardiology (ESC) established the SCORE project in the early 2000s, which developed a more accurate risk prediction tool for the European populations [224]. The European Society of Cardiology (ESC) SCORE was recalibrated later by a Greek team into the HellenicSCORE which takes into consideration the pervasiveness of cardiovascular risk factors in the Greek population [225]. This shows that a variety of CVD risk prediction tools exist with different sets of risk factors from different countries and populations, which have large variations in regard to their performance [226]. The majority of the scores use a common set of risk factors, which is known as classical and are similar to those mentioned previously such as age, gender, etc. [226], while other risk prediction tools have incorporated more advanced markers of CVD like C-reactive protein test, heart-type fatty acid binding protein, etc. [226]. The majority of the risk prediction tools are based on stochastic statistical models that consider individual variables based on cohort studies to calculate the overall risk for a future event [227]. Despite all the above-mentioned techniques for early detection of CVD by risk indication, there is still a high percentage of CVD occurrence in people without the risk factors or categories in low-to-moderate risk. Besides that, approximately 20% of the high-risk category of CVD was misjudged due to the misclassification of the risk [226]. Hence, there is a need to identify new methodologies that would improve the risk prediction of CVDs [228–231].

5.3 ARTIFICIAL INTELLIGENCE FOR DETECTION OF CVD

With today's fast-developing technology with advanced computing speeds and newer AI learning techniques, AI has been increasingly used in the application of health care [232]. AI has been incorporated in risk indication techniques in various scientific fields, including health monitoring due to the large amount of data, analytical processing, and algorithms for data manipulation [226]. The two subareas of AI are called machine learning and deep learning. Machine learning is a scientific algorithm and statistical model that is used to perform a specific task relying on the inference derived from the data. Deep learning can process a wider range of data, requires less manual preprocessing of data by humans, and can sometimes produce more accurate results compared to machine learning when trained with a sufficient amount of data. Figure 5.1 shows the summary of the core difference between machine learning and deep learning.

5.3.1 Machine Learning

Since the early 2000s, machine learning has grown in the area of health science [233], where it has been applied in various healthcare and biomedicine applications [234]. This application includes cancer prediction [235], radiology imaging [236], research on aging [237], and cardiovascular risk prediction [238]. Machine learning is a technique of learning from data, which is well-known and established by a statistical approach where the model is

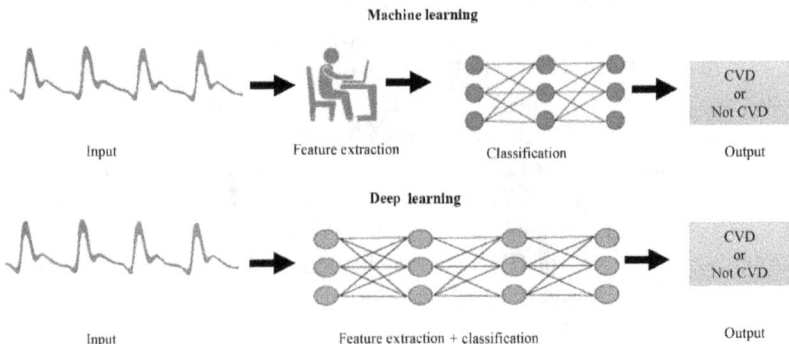

FIGURE 5.1 Machine learning versus deep learning.

built based on the data, which is a subset of a larger population [226]. For machine learning, there is a need for human intervention in each stage to build the model [239] such as manual feature extraction of data, and the efficiency of the machine learning is evaluated by the prediction performance. Currently, for CVD risk indication, machine learning techniques are built with complex models considering features from the accessible data of patient's bioclinical risk factors, socioeconomic, lifestyle, and psychological characteristics [226]. Artificial neural networks (ANNs) is a machine learning technique that has been used in current research in the area of healthcare. ANN is an arithmetic tool for pattern recognition that has been the subject of renewed research interest during the past 10 years. In 1960, Minsky [240] showed that the research in neural networks that began in the 1940s had applications to solve simple problems. Neural network research is being revived currently as learning models, which are commonly used in different network formats and learning rules. ANN is a computer system modeled on the human brain and nervous system for decision-making, and the artificial neuron is called a perceptron. Therefore, an ANN is formed by a multilayer perceptron, which is a combination of multiple perceptron's in more than one layer, as shown in Figure 5.2.

Each neuron is a sum of weighted input that transmits a transfer function to the next neuron level, which finally activates the output unit and produces the ANN output [241]. Feeding in training data and adapting the weights according to the error from network output to intended output is the process of training the ANNs. There are two types of methods, one of which is supervised learning and the other, unsupervised learning. Supervised learning techniques connect inputs to learned outputs, whereas unsupervised learning techniques are typically used for classifications of the database. A key algorithm for the weight update procedure is the introduction of the backpropagation algorithm by Rumelhart et al. [242, 243] in 1986, which is commonly used although there

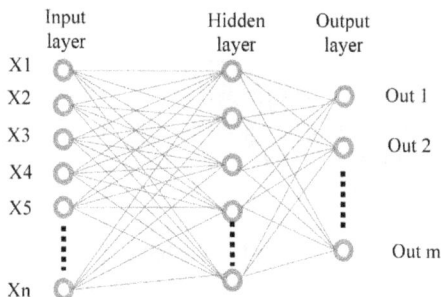

FIGURE 5.2 Multilayer perceptron.

are alternative processes, such as cascade correlation and general regression [241, 244].

In the identification of CVD, ANN is utilized in four significant cardiovascular medicinal zones, which are coronary artery disease, electrocardiography (ECG), cardiac image analysis, and cardiovascular drug dosing [164]. Numerous research [245–247] has been published that relates ANNs to diverse areas of importance to cardiovascular experts. ANNs was a contrivance by Akay [248] to diagnose coronary artery disease with a backpropagation-trained algorithm with the input data of the history of the patient, physical examination data, and preprocessed recordings of diastolic heart sound. From the research study of 63 abnormal and 37 normal subjects, the ANNs gave an output of 84% for positive prediction accuracy and 89% for negative accuracy. Itchhaporia et al. [244] have done similar research for diagnosing coronary artery disease. This research obtained 80% positive prediction accuracy and 90% negative prediction accuracy. By setting >50% obstruction of the left main coronary artery, the ANNs were trained to recognize significant coronary artery disease.

ECG can be interpreted and analyzed using computer technology [249, 250], and ANNs can be used to automate the analysis and interpretation of the ECG signals. Bortolan et al. [251] mentioned that ANNs can also be used for interpretation of ECGs to statistical analysis of conventional linear discriminant analysis and multigroup logistic discriminant analysis. Edenbrandt et al. [252] used ANNs to categorize ECG ST-T segments and compared it with clinical findings. The output of ANNs gave an 80% accuracy compared to an experienced cardiologist. Heden et al. [253] used ANNs to diagnose myocardial infarction from the analysis of the ECGs of 1,107 patients who had undergone diagnostic cardiac catheterization. This research study has compared the ANNs with the conventional automated ECG interpretation with the Glasgow program [249]. The conventional method showed a 66% sensitivity, whereas ANNs showed a 78% sensitivity. Therefore, there is only a minor difference between both approaches.

Radiofrequency catheter ablation is used as therapy for patients with cardiac arrhythmias. Before performing radiofrequency ablation, ANNs are used to focus on the accessory pathways. The trained ANN provides an output for each of the networks, which indicates the presence or absence of the accessory pathway site. After the ANN was trained manually by Dassen et al. [254] to generate data from 60 cases, 25 cases were used to test the network. Predicted locations and actual locations were exact fits for 15 cases, a border zone between two locations was predicted by the network for eight cases, and the prediction was incorrect for two other cases. ANNs could be useful in these types of studies even where causal relations between physiologic mechanisms and ECG findings are concluded by the investigators. ANNs will potentially reduce process time, decrease radiation exposure, prevent unsuccessful energy applications, and increase overall success rates by optimizing the ablation technique with the localization of an accessory pathway by preprocessing information. Recognition of lesions as benign or malignant images on mammography, hepatic ultrasound images, and avascular necrosis of the femoral head in magnetic resonance images has been trained in ANNs [250]. ANNs can be used to automate the segmentation and recognition of structures or regions of interest in echocardiographic and scintigraphy images in cardiovascular applications.

The limitation of above-mentioned techniques of utilizing ANNs for CVD detection is that they cannot be incorporated for 24-h monitoring, as the technique of acquiring the data is by Holter monitoring or one time measurement. Hence, ANNs using blood pressure data would be ideal as in today's technology era where there are ambulatory medical devices that could acquire the blood pressure readings noninvasively such as SphygmoCorCVMS, AtCor Medical, Australia [108, 119, 120] and BPro + A-Pulse, HealthSTATS [108–110]. Many researchers are working in the field of CVD prediction utilizing blood pressure data with other additional information such as chronic risk factors (diabetes, obesity, smoking, etc), psychobehavior (physical activity, sleep quality, respiration, stress, depression, etc), genome (family history) and others [255]. An ANN-based system that utilizes 24-h blood pressure monitor input to diagnose and analyze therapeutic interventions for ambulatory hypertensive patients named "Hypernet" was developed by Poll et al. [247]. The therapeutic recommendations of Hypernet were tested against those of an experienced specialist for a test set of 35 patients. The output showed that Hypernet achieved a sensitivity of 92% and a specificity of 96% when evaluated for both diagnosis and treatment ability. The Self-applied Questionnaire (SAQ) study to predict CVD proposed by Shen et al. [256] was utilized, where the study was based on the analysis of the common risk features of the disease and other data information by the SAQ. The study was based on blood pressure, smoking, blood cholesterol, sex, and age to determine the risk of having CVD. The study utilized an ANN, which is a multilayered feedforward neural network with the backpropagation method. The outcome of the ANN was a 67% accuracy for the detection. A hybrid system constructed by genetic algorithm and ANN was proposed by Amin et al. [257] to predict CVD based on risk factor. Amin et al. [257] highlighted the two major disadvantages of the algorithm, which are: it is impossible to find the initial weights that are globally optimized, and the algorithm takes a lot of time to converge. To address these disadvantages, these researchers applied a genetic algorithm to optimize the weights of the ANNs, which gave a better performance than the basic ANN, which resulted in 96.2% accuracy for training and 89% accuracy for testing. Sonawane and Patil [258] developed an ANN trained by vector quantization algorithm using random order incremental training to predict CVD. The input layer of the ANN consists of 13 neurons, which are the clinical features of CVD dataset, and the output layer was a single neuron, which shows the presence or absence of CVD. The output is set to a single neuron to obtain less error and high accuracy. The performance of the ANN is improved by training the network with a higher number of epochs, where the obtained accuracy was 85.55%. Other than ANNs, a hybrid machine learning model based on decision tree, support vector machine, and Naïve Bayes was proposed by Bashir et al. [259]. This research utilized different classifiers to obtain the majority voting scheme, where the scheme works in two different steps. The first step is the three classifiers output results, and the second step combines the decisions of the three classifiers output to develop a new model created by the majority voting scheme. The approach attained a 74% sensitivity, 82% accuracy, and 83% specificity for the prediction of CVD. Feshki and Shijani [260] developed a model on CVD prediction by using feature selections and classification for a specific dataset. The developed model operates by partitioning the dataset into subsets (sick and healthy people) and identifying the subset having the highest accuracy using particle swarm optimization with a feed-forward backpropagation algorithm as a classifier. From the outcome of the model, it is known that the feature selection and backpropagation feed-forward neural network with particle swarm optimization is an effective method, as it was able to give 91.94% accurate results.

These studies illustrate the potential of ANNs in blood pressure monitoring wearable devices, as they can continuously monitor the blood pressure reading and incorporate risk factors of CVDs such as age, gender, smoking habits, obesity, etc. However, these studies with ANNs or machine learning techniques that utilize history and physical examination data such as obesity are just an indication of risk but cannot be relied on as a predictive indicator for CVD. For example, despite obesity being a strong independent CVD predictor even in the absence of other risk factors, the clinical outcome is not linear for a relationship between higher BMI and the onset of CVD [261]. The assumption of excess body mass (obesity) as a lead to CVD is not necessarily accurate because there are studies showing the potential of protective effects of obesity when it coexists with CVD, where this phenomenon is called obesity paradox [262–264]. This paradox has been investigated with heart failure and coronary heart disease [261], and recently, research data has also shown that this paradox applies to hypertension [265, 266], atrial fibrillation [267, 268], pulmonary arterial hypertension [269], and congenital heart disease [270]. As for blood pressure monitoring, the readings of systolic and diastolic are normally a good indicator for hypertension. Despite hypertension being a leading risk factor for premature death worldwide [271] which typically relates to cardiovascular risk, there are many generated debates and editorial commentaries [272–274] in regard to hypertension being an indicator for CVD. Therefore, there is a need to use the entire blood pressure pulse as training for machine learning, rather than just the systolic and diastolic values to give a better detection of CVD. By feeding the entire blood pressure pulse waveform into an AI, the waveform's morphology change can be used to determine CVD. The blood pressure waveform is a fusion of the forward waveform generated by left ventricular ejection and a reverse/backward traveling reflected waveform caused by the sites of impedance mismatch, for example, the arterial taper and difference in vessel stiffness, which often occur at bifurcations [275, 276]. The impedance change generates numerous reflected 'wavelets' which are summed together to produce the effective reflected wave, which results in the increase of the systolic pressure in the central arteries and also produces the features in the blood pressure waveform such as the notch. Other than the systolic pressure being an indicator for hypertension resulting in cardiovascular events, the feature of the blood pressure waveform can be used to indicate cardiovascular events. For example, the notch, which is one of the blood pressure waveform features, is the primary signal that facilitates the endothelial-to- mesenchymal transformation during cardiac valve formation. The endothelium is conceivably one of the largest organ systems, and research on its diversity and the multiplex functions it performs continues to emerge. Significant evidence has implicated 'endothelial dysfunction' as a contributing factor to a number of CVDs [277]. To feed the entire blood pressure waveform into an AI, the blood pressure waveform would need a feature extractor to extract the features of the signal. However, the extraction of features is a laborious task [278] and would need a tremendous amount of information to identify the features that are related to CVD. Hence, by utilizing deep learning, the feature extraction can be automated without the need for manual extraction, as the deep learning model would identify the key features of the signal and relate them to signal classification.

5.3.2 Deep Learning

Deep learning originated from the study of ANNs, which are computational models inspired by biological neural networks in human brains, which have been extensively studied since the 1980s [279]. The idea of the implementation of deep learning is inspired by biological processes, powered by high-performance computing hardware, which has made very deep models computationally practicable for a real-world application. For example, in the convolutional neural network (CNN), the connectivity between neurons reassembles the network of neurons in the animal/human visual cortex [280]. Deep learning models have achieved superior results compared to other high-end machine learning models and even compared to human experts in many applied areas in recent years [279]. Furthermore, in recent years of research

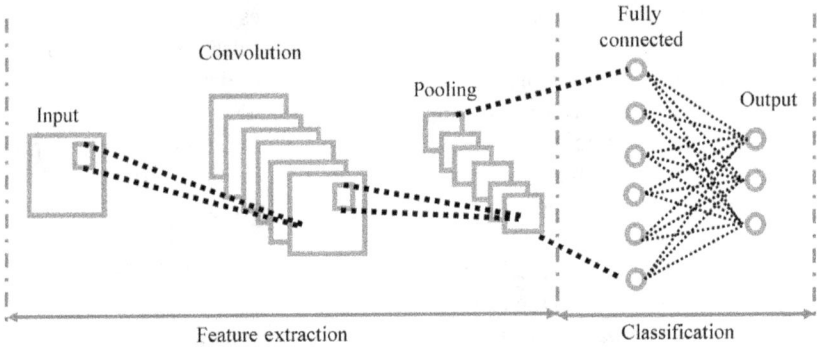

FIGURE 5.3   A typical convolutional neural network architecture.

and development in deep learning, various neural network's structures have been designed for signal processing. Recurrent neural network [281] is a deep learning model based on internal memory where it is used to process arbitrary time series input sequences such as speech recognition, handwriting recognition, etc. Long short-term memory [282], another deep learning model, can effectively prevent the occurrence of gradient vanishing from processing time series signals. The most remarkable achievements in recent years for pattern/feature classification using deep learning are done using CNNs [283–287]. CNNs provide an end-to-end learning model where a trained CNN by the gradient descent method can learn the characteristics of the input data and further complete the pattern classification [288–301]. CNN has a very strong ability to learn the features and pattern classification because the features of the lower layers are derived from the partial information and convolutional kernel with shared weights from the upper layer [283]. In the field of biomedical engineering, as in biomedical signal analysis, the entire blood pressure pulse waveform was utilized in training deep learning models. CNN is the ideal deep learning method as it mimics the visual of the human's neuron network interpreting the entire signal with regard to the signal's features to relate to the CVD. A typical CNN consists of a number of convolutional layers, pooling layers, and fully connected layers as its hidden layers, as shown in Figure 5.3.

In recent years, CNN has been used for the classification of human physiological signal patterns such as ECG, phonocardiogram (PCG), and blood pressure waveform. Table 5.1 shows some of the recent work of using the ECG signal for classification/detection. For PCG, there are researchers who utilized the Aalborg University heart sounds database from PhysioNet/Computing in Cardiology Challenge 2016 to verify the developed algorithms for classification of normal and abnormal heart sound recordings using CNN, as shown in

TABLE 5.1 Convolutional neural network (CNN) using electrocardiogram (ECG)

REFERENCES	DETECTION	METHOD	ACCURACY (%)
[288]	Arrhythmia	Nonlinear transform for R-peak detection and a 1D CNN with a variable learning rate	92.7
[289]	Arrhythmia	Wavelet transform (WT) for denoising and R-peak detection and a two-layer 1D CNN	97.5
[290]	Arrhythmia	Denoising filters, Pan–Tomkins, AlexNet for feature extraction and PCA for classification	92.0
[291]	Arrhythmia	34-layer CNN to classify the ECG signals into 14 types of output classes	80
[292]	Arrhythmia	11-layer CNN with the output layer of four neurons, each representing the normal (Nsr), Afib, Afl, and Vfib ECG class	92.5
[293]	Myocardial infarction	CNN for the automated detection of a normal and MI ECG beats (with noise and without noise)	93.53, 95.22
[294]	Coronary artery disease	Using different durations (two- and five-seconds durations) of ECG segments with CNN	94.95, 95.11
[295]	Atrial fibrillation	Multiscale CNN (AFDB, LTAFDB, private)	98.18
[296]	Abnormal ECG	Identify abnormal ECG using lead-CNN and rule inference	86.22
[297]	Arrhythmia	Active learning and a two-layer CNN fed with ECG and RR interval	Multiple [nearly 100% accuracy in normal and ventricular ectopic beat predictions]

(*continued*)

TABLE 5.1 (Continued)

REFERENCES	DETECTION	METHOD	ACCURACY (%)
[298]	Atrial fibrillation	CNN with spectrograms from short time Fourier transform or stationary WT (AFDB)	98.29
[299]	Congestive heart failure	11-layer CNN model for CHF diagnosis	98.97
[300]	ST event	Classify ST events from ECG using transfer learning on Inception v3	0.867
[301]	Fetal ECG segments	Three-layer CNN for classifying fetal ECG segments	77.85
[302]	Arrhythmia	Attention-based time-incremental CNN, achieving both spatial and temporal fusion of information from ECG signals	81.2%
[303]	Heart disease	Automatic ECG diagnosis using CNN to detect normal, atrial premature beat and premature ventricular contraction for the classification of heart disease.	98.33
[304]	Arrhythmia	Continuous wavelet transform (CWT) is used to decompose ECG signals to obtain different time-frequency components, and CNN is used to extract features from the 2D-scalogram composed of the above time-frequency components	98.74

TABLE 5.2   Convolutional neural network (CNN) using phonocardiogram (PCG)

REFERENCE	METHOD	ACCURACY (%)
[305]	124 time-frequency features were extracted as the input to a variant of the AdaBoost classifier, and a second classifier using CNN was trained using PCGs cardiac cycles decomposed into four frequency bands. The outputs were combined with the decision rule from both AdaBoost and CNN	86.02
[306]	Filtered by using Windowed-sinc Hamming filter algorithm to remove signals regarded as noise. The filtered recordings are then scaled and segmented. Using the filtered and segmented recordings, a four-layer CNN was trained to extract features and construct a classification function	79.5
[307]	Two-layer CNN and Mel-frequency cepstral coefficients for automatic classification of heart sound	83.99
[308]	Spectrogram by extracting a set of time-frequency parameters to be fed into a five-layer CNN with dropout	91.6
[309]	Spectrogram by segmenting and preprocessing by using the neuromorphic auditory sensor to decompose the audio information into frequency bands to feed into the CNN which has a modified AlexNet	94.16

Table 5.2. The database consists of five databases labelled from A to E that contain 3126 PCG recordings, with recordings lasting from 5 to 120 seconds.

On the other hand, for blood pressure waveforms, Hu et al. [310] utilized Shannon Energy Envelope, Hilbert Transform (SEEHT) and a CNN to classify the blood pressure pulse waveform into health and subhealth. The outcome of the research shows a 72.31% accuracy on classification of health against subhealth and a 96.33% accuracy on arteriosclerosis against nonarteriosclerosis. This research also shows that TCM doctors are able to identify health for about 60% using pulse wave because the effective features for classification are uncertain [310]. This shows that the CNN performs better in feature identification and classifying the blood pressure pulse signal compared to a human.

Moon et al. [311] applied arterial blood pressure waveform data recorded from liver transplantation surgeries to the CNN to estimate stroke volume (SV) which attained a concordance rate of 74.15% during surgery. Shimazaki et al. investigated CNN on photoplethysmography signals based on the relationship between pulse waveform and blood pressure reading. The pulse wave and blood pressure data were collected from 78 subjects to conduct a precision assessment experiment where the CNN was able to attain a correlation coefficient (R) of 0.71 compared to using conventional methods (geometric features + multiple regression analysis) which attained a 0.63 correlation coefficient [312]. In addition, Li et al. [283] utilized a CNN model to identify a one-to-one pulse pattern to its corresponding CVD. In the study by Li et al., five CVDs and complications were extracted from medical records for the first CNN classifier and four physiological parameters related to selected diseases were also extracted to build the second CNN classifier. The outcome of each CNN was able to attain 95% and 89% accuracy for the first and second CNN, respectively [283]. From these research areas, it is known that the diversity of pulse wave morphology results in difficulty in pulse-based diagnosis especially in pulse waveform pattern classification. Nevertheless, from the above findings, it is known that CNN is a promising method that can be utilized for pulse waveform pattern classification, and it outperforms the conventional methods in pattern classification due to its ability to extract informative features. Furthermore, the majority of CNN [283–287] models are used for pattern/feature classification, but this does not indicate risk or act as a predictive role.

Hence, to attain a risk indication-based CNN for future implementation in a predictive role, the output must be based on a numerical regressive outcome where the input of the CNN would be a full physiological signal waveform and the output would be a numerical number rather than a classifier. By having the numerical output for CNN, this technique can mimic the conventional technique of risk assessment, similar to how it was conducted for indicating the risk for hypertension. For example, the numerical reading of blood pressure over a time of 24 hours is considered healthy if the blood pressure reading is in the range between 90/60 and 120/80 mmHg and if the blood pressure reading is in the range of 140/90 mmHg or higher, it would be high blood pressure, which is a risk indication for hypertension. Therefore, to develop a pulse waveform pattern regression based on CNN to attain a numerical output, there is a need for input data of blood pressure pulse waveform and its corresponding numerical output. This can be attained, as in today's research world cardiovascular models are available, where the inputs of the models are numerical values, and the output is the corresponding blood pressure waveform.

Cardiovascular System Models

6

Modeling of the cardiovascular system was first done to study the circulation of blood in the human body. By studying the blood circulation of the human body using cardiovascular models, conceptual ideas can be tested out before proceeding to clinical trials. Harvey announced the discovery of the cardiovascular system in the 17th century by denoting the heart as the pump of the cardiovascular system [313]. The model sets the blood flow in a unidirectional flow in a closed-loop circuit through systemic and pulmonary circulations [314]. Modeling starts by doing a mathematical model of the cardiovascular system. The equation for each part of the cardiovascular system is identified, and all the equations are then combined to form a full equation for the cardiovascular system. The mathematical model uses basic fluid dynamic equations, especially Navier–Stokes equations. Poiseuille's flow and Reynolds number play a big part in determining the mathematical model of the cardiovascular system. The lower the Reynolds number, the higher the viscosity of the blood. The equation is then placed into a computational simulation, which is known as a fluid–structure interaction (FSI) model so that the unknown parameters can be altered using an iterative method to know the effect of the parameters on the cardiovascular system. In the FSI model, the density of blood is set to be 1.03 g/cm^3 and wall density is set to 1.2 g/cm^3. The FSI model can be converted to a 3D model, and then to a 1D and finally to a simplified 0D model. In the 3D model, a Navier–Stokes equation is coupled with a structural model for the vessel wall. On the other hand, in the 1D model, a net of systems of hyperbolic equations is used to determine mean pressure and flow rate. The 0D model uses a system of algebra-ordinary differential equations, which is often nonlinear to determine the mean pressure and flow rate in time [315–322]. By comparing all the 3D, 1D, and 0D models in Table 6.1, it is reasonably justified to use the 0D model as the model for overall cardiovascular blood circulation analysis to detect cardiovascular disease because it is comprehensively simple, requires less computational effort, and the model covers the whole cardiovascular circulation system, which analyses the overall pressure, volume, and flow of the

TABLE 6.1 Summarized comparison of various computational cardiovascular models

MODEL	TYPE OF PARAMETER MODEL	TYPE OF FLOW DISTRIBUTION	TYPES OF GOVERNING EQUATIONS	APPLICATIONS OF MODEL
0-D	Lumped	Uniform	Ordinary differential equation (ODE) for conservation of mass and momentum and algebraic equilibrium equation to convert volume to pressure	Appropriate for analysis of pressure, flow, and volume of blood distribution in system. Can, at times, give boundary conditions for three-dimensional models
1-D	Distributed	Nonuniform	Partial differential equation (PDE) of conservation of mass and momentum, and equilibrium equations	Appropriate for analyzation of reflection or transmission impact, which permits better boundary conditions for three-dimensional models
2-D	Distributed	Nonuniform	Partial differential equation (PDE) of conservation of mass and momentum, and equilibrium equations	Appropriate for analysis on the change of velocity in an axisymmetric tube which permits better boundary conditions for three-dimensional models with certain limits of applicability
3-D	Distributed	Nonuniform	Partial differential equation (PDE) of conservation of mass and momentum, and equilibrium equations	Appropriate for analysis of complex flow patterns in small regions of the cardiovascular circulatory system

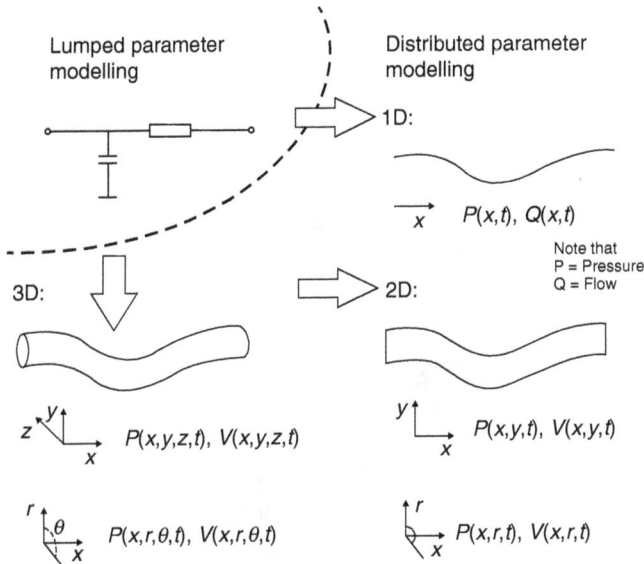

FIGURE 6.1   Different scales of modeling.

blood. Figure 6.1 shows all the scales of the 3D, 2D, and 1D modeling from the 0D model.

6.1 ZERO DIMENSIONAL

For modeling a 0D model, the concept of hydraulic-electrical analog is often used. The 0D model relates the blood flow circulation to electric conduction in a circuit. Blood flow follows the law of mass conservation, which uses Poiseuille's law for steady-state momentum equilibrium and Navier–Stokes law for unsteady-state momentum balance, which in the analogy is similar to an electric circuit, which uses Ohm's law for steady-state voltage–current relation and Kirchhoff's law for current balance. The electrical circuit has a resistor, capacitor, and inductance, which correlate with a cardiovascular system. Inductance represents inertance, which is the measure of the pressure difference in a fluid due to the change in blood flow rate over time. Capacitance represents compliance which is the measure of the change in blood volume when subjected to an applied force. Resistance represents the peripheral resistance in the vessels of the blood flow in the cardiovascular system [324].

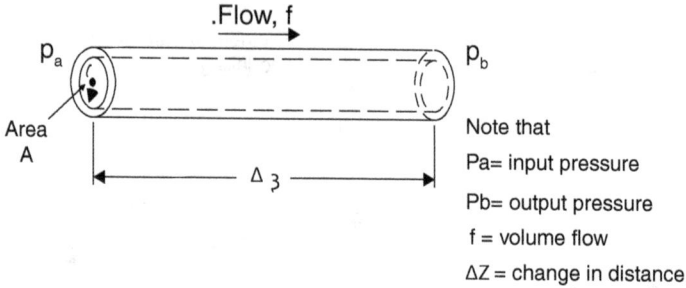

FIGURE 6.2 Idealized segment of a vein or artery.

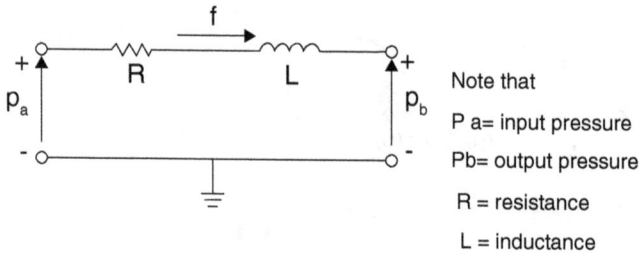

FIGURE 6.3 Equivalent lumped fluid-flow circuit, ignoring wall compliance.

Figure 6.2 is a 3D model, which is converted to its 0D model as shown in Figure 6.3. In Figure 6.3, R and L are used to model resistance and represent the wall inertia, respectively. The change of pressure from p_a (input pressure) to p_b (output pressure) can be discovered in Equation 6.1.

$$(p_a - p_b)|vis = f * R \tag{6.1}$$

For this Equation 6.1, it is assumed that flow is uniform across the vein or artery where the volume flow rate is f.

The mass of the blood flow can be determined by Equation 6.2.

$$M = \rho * A * \Delta Z \tag{6.2}$$

where ρ is blood density, A is the cross-sectional area of the vessel, and ΔZ is the change of length of the vessel for Equation 6.2. Blood flow velocity (v) across the vessel radius is assumed to be uniform, whereby the total flow is given as

$$f = v * A. \tag{6.3}$$

The second law of motion rule in Newton relates to the behavior of objects for which all existing forces are not balanced. This second law states that the acceleration of an object is dependent upon two variables, which are the net force acting upon the object and the mass of the object. In this case, Newton's second law is used to drive the force needed to balance the acceleration of blood using Equation 6.3

$$M(dv/dt) = (\rho * A * \Delta z) * (d(f/A)/dt) = (\rho * \Delta z) * df/dt \qquad (6.4)$$

This acceleration force must be equal to the acceleration at the pressure difference at the end of the cross-sectional area of the vein or artery. Hence, the pressure differences between p_a and p_b are multiplied with the cross-sectional area of the vein or artery using Newton's second law of motion.

$$(p_a - p_b) * A \qquad (6.5)$$

To obtain the acceleration part of the pressure drop equation of

$$(p_a - p_b)|accel = (\rho * \Delta z/A) * df/dt \qquad (6.6)$$

Inertance is the coefficient of the flow derivative in this equation, resulting in

$$l = \rho * \Delta z/A \qquad (6.7)$$

The resistance of flow is obtained by using Poiseuille's steady-state formula which is given as

$$R = 8 * \pi * \mu * \Delta z/A \qquad (6.8)$$

Therefore, the pressure drop is equated to the sum of the viscous resistance and mass of acceleration, which is

$$p_a - p_b = f * R + l * df/dt \qquad (6.9)$$

In fact, velocity is lower near the wall of the vessel, with an overall parabolic cross section of the flow velocities, which gives a slightly better value for the inertance based on a two-radial segment approximation, resulting in

$$l = 9 * \rho * \Delta z/4 * A = 9 * \rho * \Delta z/(4 * \pi * r^2) \qquad (6.10)$$

Compliance of a cylindrical vessel shows the elasticity of the wall, which results in

$$C = 3*\pi*r3*\Delta z/2*E*h \tag{6.11}$$

where the radius is r, the length is Δz, wall thickness is h, and young bulk modulus of elasticity, E. The wall material is uniform with a Poisson ratio of

$$\sigma = 1/2. \tag{6.12}$$

When the fluid velocity is zero, pressure through the vessel is pa. Meanwhile, q is the total volume of the segment, and qu is the unstressed volume when transmural pressure is zero.

$$q = qu + pa * C \tag{6.13}$$

Compliance may be determined by varying pa by Δpa in $q = qu + pa * c$ by observing diameter and the volume change rather than using Equation 6.14 as E and h are usually unavailable because it will not be practical to obtain them from a living being. Compliance is found by

$$C = \Delta q/\Delta pa. \tag{6.14}$$

Compliance has a limited range of positive transmural pressure. This is to ensure that the vessel walls would not reach their limit of expansion and result in vessel rupture [127].

A complete 0D cardiovascular circulatory system by Korakianitis and Shi which shows the human cardiovascular system in the simplest form, where the schematic of the model was extracted from Shi et al.'s model in the CellML model repository. This 0D cardiovascular circulation model can be regarded as a limited representation of a 1D model [325]. The model is made up of three main parts, which are the heart, systemic loop, and pulmonary loop. The model divides the heart model with chambers exactly like the human heart, and diodes are used as valves to ensure the flow is in one direction. The systemic loop is modeled with five main parts, which are systemic aortic sinus, systemic artery, systemic arteriole, systemic capillary, and systemic vein. Same as the systemic loop, the pulmonary loop is modeled with five main parts, which are pulmonary aortic sinus, pulmonary artery, pulmonary arteriole, pulmonary capillary, and pulmonary vein. The systemic aortic sinus, systemic artery, pulmonary aortic sinus, and the pulmonary artery are modeled as RLC components. Moreover, systemic arteriole, systemic capillary, pulmonary arteriole, and pulmonary capillary are modeled as resistors. Finally, the systemic vein and pulmonary vein are modeled as RC components like the

TABLE 6.2 Electrical equivalence of parameters in blood flow model by T. Korakianitis and Y. Shi

SYMBOL	PARAMETER	ELECTRICAL EQUIVALENT
P	Pressure	Voltage
Q	Flow	Current
R	Resistance	Resistance
C	Compliance	Capacitance
L	Inertance	Inductance

TABLE 6.3 Cardiovascular system described by parameters in blood flow model by T. Korakianitis and Y. Shi

SYMBOL	PARAMETER	CARDIOVASCULAR SYSTEM
R	Resistance	Frictional loss
C	Compliance	Wall elasticity
L	Inertance	Blood inertia
E	Elastance	Wall stiffness
CV	Flow coefficient	Blood flow through valves

Windkessel model [325]. For this model, the parameters related to electrical equivalents, such as pressure, flow, resistance, compliance, and inertance, are represented by the voltage, current, resistance, capacitance, and inductance in the circuit, respectively. Table 6.2 shows the parameters represented by its electrical equivalent in the circuit.

Table 6.2 can also be used to relate the body's cardiovascular system to give the correlation between the electrical equivalents and the human body's cardiovascular system. Table 6.3 shows the parameters represented by its cardiovascular system.

There are three templates (TempR, TempRC, and TempRLC), which were defined to provide zero-dimensional representations of the linearized governing equations for pressure and flow in the vessel segments to establish the relationships between P, Q, R, L, and C components at the input to express the output. The TempR defines the relationship between pressure and flow, whereas the TempRC defines the first derivative of the input pressure in terms of flow and capacitance. Meanwhile, the TempRLC defines the first derivative of the output flow, which shows the relationship between the R, L, and C components. Table 6.4 shows the equations that were obtained from the 'Mathematics' section of Shi et al.'s CellML model in the CellML model repository [326].

TABLE 6.4   The relationship between the model parameters and TempR, TempRC, and TempRLC equations, respectively

COMPONENTS	EQUATIONS
TempR	$P_{in} = P_{out} + RQ_{in}$ $Q_{out} = Q_{in}$
TempRC	$\dfrac{d}{dt}\left(P_{in}\right) = \dfrac{Q_{in} - Q_{out}}{C}$ $Q_{out} = \dfrac{P_{in} - P_{out}}{R}$
TempRLC	$\dfrac{d}{dt}\left(P_{in}\right) = \dfrac{Q_{in} - Q_{out}}{C}$ $\dfrac{d}{dt}\left(Q_{out}\right) = \dfrac{P_{in} - P_{out} - RQ_{out}}{L}$

This complete 0D cardiovascular circulatory system by Korakianitis and Shi can simulate pressure, flow, and volume of blood and generates results, which are satisfactory given its simplicity. However, the downside of the 0D model is its inability to simulate the nonlinear convective acceleration term compared to its 1D model.

Pressure flow components of the model obey the same fundamental equations as the electrical circuit equivalent referring to Table 6.4, for example:

$$P = R \times F \quad V = R \times F \tag{6.15}$$

$$P = L*dF/dt \quad V = L*dI/dt \tag{6.16}$$

$$P = Q/C \quad V = Q/C \tag{6.17}$$

$$F = dQ/dt \quad I = dQ/dt \tag{6.18}$$

The compliances in this model are modeled linearly with unstressed volumes. Equation 6.19 sums of the volume of stressed and unstressed are as shown.

$$Qn = Qnu + Qns \tag{6.19}$$

Volume at a node in this model is defined as Equation 6.20 of this model (0 to t):

$$Qn = \int (F_{in} - F_{out})dt + Q_n(0) \tag{6.20}$$

The pressure is calculated from the stressed volume using Equation 6.21 of this model:

$$P = Q_{ns}/C_n = (Q_n - Q_{nu})/C_n \qquad (6.21)$$

This complete 0D cardiovascular circulatory system by Vincent Rideout generates results, which are satisfactory even though it does not include baroreceptor sensor connections to the central nervous system. Besides that, despite the model being uncontrolled, it is stable due to the Frank–Starling mechanism. Pressure, flow, and volume of the blood can be simulated using this model.

In a nutshell, the Vincent Rideout model represents a real human cardiovascular system with more insight, whereas the model by Korakianitis and Shi is too simplified. Moreover, Vincent Rideout model has more parameters than Korakianitis and Shi's model, which can be helpful in studying and diagnosing cardiovascular diseases. This is because each parameter would relate to each output of time in the signal. The computational time and complexity are also well balanced in Vincent Rideout model. On top of that, end-diastolic pressure, initial flow, and unstressed volumes of the blood vessels are also provided by Vincent Rideout. Should these values be obtained via clinical study, it would have been time-consuming. So, this model presents an advantage in terms of time as well. Furthermore, Vincent Rideout model has 36 different dynamic parameters, which consist of 16 resistance parameters, 12 compliance parameters, and eight inductance parameters. All the parameters' default values are given to form a healthy patient output signal. The Vincent Rideout model can produce four main output signals, which are right ventricular pressure (PRV), the pulmonary artery pressure (PPV), the left ventricular pressure (PLV), and the aortic pressure (PA1). The aortic pressure (PA1) can be used to study the feature of the signal that coincides with the cardiovascular disease signal, as aortic signal is common for medical experts to determine the patient's heart condition.

6.2 One Dimensional

One-dimensional (1D) model is developed using the simplified Navier–Stokes equations which represent the pressure and flow at any point of the blood vessel of the cardiovascular system [327–329]. With a large amount of computation, a 1D model can be used to represent the phenomenon of blood pressure wave propagation. The common applications of 1D model are simulation of pulse wave propagation dynamics [330–336], wave intensity analysis [337–339], estimation of central aortic pressure [340–343], and assessing the performance of algorithms and indexes [344–346]. The blood in the cardiovascular system is assumed to be an incompressible Newtonian fluid, and the vessel is an axisymmetric cylindrical tube for a 1D model. Hence, the 1D model is governed by two equations, which are the continuity equation and momentum equation [347]. Both these equations describe the motion of the blood flow in the vessel and contraction and expansion of the vessel's wall during blood flow. Equation 6.22 is the continuity equation, and Equation 6.23 is the momentum equation, where q is the blood flow rate, x is the distance along the vessel, A is the cross-sectional area of the blood vessel, t is time taken for the flow, ρ is the blood density, p is the blood pressure, r is the vessel radius, and μ is the viscosity.

$$\partial q/\partial x = \partial A/\partial t \tag{6.22}$$

$$\partial q/\partial t + 4/3 * \partial(q^2/A)/\partial x = -(A/\rho)*(\partial p/\partial x) - (8\mu/\rho r^2)*q \tag{6.23}$$

For solving a 1D model using the Navier–Stokes equations, there are two types of domain methods, which are time domain and frequency domain. In the time domain, the method can solve for linear and nonlinear equations.

However, the frequency domain can only solve linear equations. The Navier–Stokes equations for 1D model are generally nonlinear where they are solved in the time domain using numerical methods. There are many numerical methods for solving the partial differential equation of Navier–Stokes such as the method of characteristics, finite difference method, finite volume method, finite element method, and spectral method. It is very complicated to utilize the method of characteristics to solve the differential equation, which has three independent variables, and there may still be problems to be solved. By using the method of characteristics, the governing equations can be solved [348–350]. The finite difference method is used for solving complex partial differential equations. The complex partial differential equations are solved by approximating the derivatives with finite differences. In addition, the finite volume method is created from the finite difference method, where the area of calculation is focused on the series of control volumes, and there is a control volume at the surrounding of each grid point. This control volume is integrated, and a set of discrete equations are formed where they need to be solved. The finite volume method needs a high computing speed and low requirements for the grid. This method is commonly used for computations of fluid, and recently, this method can also be used to solve differential equations [351, 352]. On the other hand, the spectral method is a method that uses an orthogonal function or intrinsic function with a class of computing techniques to solve certain differential equations, where this method is able to obtain a higher precision using fewer grid points. However, the weakness of this method is that it has poor stability and high complexity in setting the boundary conditions. This method had been used by several researchers to resolve the 1D model's pulse wave propagation equations [353, 354].

In the frequency domain method, a transmission line method is utilized to solve the Navier–Stokes equations in order to minimize the complexity of the nonlinear 1D Navier–Stokes equations by linearizing them. This method transforms hemodynamic equations into their electrical analogs, where mechanical and geometric properties of blood vessels determine the electrical parameters. $C = dA/dp = (3\pi*r^3)/2Eh$ is the capacitance (E is the Young's modulus, and h is the arterial wall thickness), $L = \rho/A = \rho/\pi*r^2$ is the inductance, and $R = 8\mu/\pi*r^4$ is the resistance [355]. The resulting equations describe the relationship between blood flow and pressure, analogous to electrical transmission line equations in a circuit. By utilizing circuit-solving techniques, these equations are efficiently addressed, reducing computational burden. The governing equations for hemodynamics and their electrical counterparts are Equations 6.24 and 6.25, where q represents blood flow and p represents pressure. These equations can be directly mapped to electrical circuit equations, facilitating efficient numerical solutions in cardiovascular modeling.

$$- \partial q/\partial x + C*(\partial p/\partial t) = 0 \qquad (6.24)$$

$$- \partial p/\partial x = L*(\partial q/\partial t) + Rq \qquad (6.25)$$

6.3 MULTISCALE

Multiscale models are a combination of 3D, 2D, 1D, and 0D to form a complex model of the cardiovascular system. The 2D and 3D models are mostly based on the Navier–Stokes equations, which are nonlinear partial differential equations. The model behavior may be parabolic, hyperbolic, or elliptic, which depends on the specific study. These models can provide detailed information on the blood flow in the vessel, where the model describes the hemodynamic phenomena in a specific region of the cardiovascular system. The 2D models are usually utilized to describe the change of blood flow velocity of the radial vessel in an axisymmetric tube [356, 357]. On the other hand, the 3D models are generally utilized to simulate and study the interaction between blood flow and the vascular walls [358, 359]. 2D and 3D models need a great amount of computational resources since they provide detailed pressure and velocity distribution in a certain vessel segment of the cardiovascular system using the concept of computational fluid dynamics. Furthermore, a multiscale model needs special attention as it is required to handle all the boundary conditions to ensure the desired output of the model is obtained mathematically. This is because one boundary condition is needed for each part of the blood vessel parameters, which interlinks with the next part of the blood vessel to form a proper blood flow in the cardiovascular circulatory system. Hence, to establish a multiscale model such as a 3D model of the whole cardiovascular system, it would need complex geometrical and mechanical information, which results in massive computational complexity. It would not be practical to be done. However, by using a multiscale model with segments of 3D or 2D with another model such as 1D or 0D, this would be possible. For example, a 3D model of a ventricular blood flow merged with a 0D model for the rest of the cardiovascular circulatory system was done by Watanabe et al. [360], where the 0D model was able to provide the pressure values as the boundary conditions for the 3D model. Similarly, Migliavacca et al. [361] merged a 3D model of a systemic to pulmonary flow in a 0D model of multiple branched circulation system model. The 0D model was used to calculate the total sum of static and kinetic pressure, which was used as the boundary condition for the upstream interface of the 3D model, and for the downstream interface, the static pressure of the 0D model was used as the boundary condition. In addition, a 0D model of a vessel network was used by Vigono-Clementel et al. [362] as terminal loads to a complex 3D model of arterial branching where the 0D model was supplied with the pressure flow rate relation to obtain the impedance values for the 3D model's boundary condition. On the other hand, a 1D model was merged by Formaggia et al. [363] with a 3D model to remove the effect of the outgoing pressure waves and reduce computational complexity when analysis of blood flow was done in regard to the compliance of the vessels. A variational approach and a Lagrange multiplier approach are the two approaches proposed by Formaggia et al. [317, 364] to derive the variable distributions at the model interface. These approaches were further elaborated by Formaggia et al. to be utilized for transient flow problems, which was implemented by Vigono-Clementel et al. [362] for the model interfaces. Hence, to obtain a cardiovascular system model by minimizing the computational complexity using multiscale is possible by combining two or more models such as a combination of 3D or 2D models, which are high-dimensional models with lower dimensional models such as 1D and 0D models.

Conclusion and Future Recommendations

7

Various studies have been done using aortic signals to detect cardiovascular diseases. Evidently, arterial pressure is the result of an interaction between the heart and the arterial system. The magnitude and shape of this pressure pulse, which is the aortic signal, will be affected by changes in the peripheral circulation or alterations in cardiac function. Hence, this is how the changes in the aortic signal relate to cardiovascular disease. However, to obtain an aortic signal, a patient has to undergo catheterization techniques. Therefore, monitoring the heart using aortic signals requires an invasive method to be performed [365, 366].

Yubing et al. have done a review on categories of 0D and 1D models. In the review, the advantages and disadvantages of 0D and 1D models are highlighted, thus providing guidance on the selection of models to assist various cardiovascular modelling studies. It also identifies directions for further development, as well as current challenges in the wider use of these models, including service to represent boundary conditions for local 3D models and translation to the clinical application [318]. By the review, it is well known that it is possible to study the aortic signal to identify its corresponding heart diseases. For example, Vincent Rideout's model has 36 different dynamic parameters, which consist of 16 resistance parameters, 12 compliance parameters, and 8 inductance parameters [324]. To form a healthy patient output signal, all the parameters default value are given. Since the healthy patient output signal is known, a study of the parameter values of this model is done in this research to obtain all the parameter values and its corresponding aortic signal. These significant values will be essential to studying cardiovascular disease signals.

There are many sensors that have been developed in today's world to acquire radial signals for monitoring. Sharmila et al. has done research on diagnosing diseases through pulse using a pressure sensor. The research objective was to obtain a radial pulse wave signal from the wrist and relate it to the

DOI: 10.1201/9781003629832-7

Indian traditional method of diagnosis. The Indian traditional method takes the pulse from the wrist by using three fingertips. The three pulses are called kappa, pitta, and vata. Therefore, three pressure transducers were attached at the wrist to obtain the three pulses [367]. In addition, Suket et al. had used a pressure sensor to obtain a radial pulse wave signal. The work was mainly on obtaining a wrist pulse acquisition and recording system. The pressure sensor, which was used for this project was MPXM2053D piezo-resistive pressure sensor. Moreover, ARM Cortex M4 architecture was used for digitization of signals and fed into the LCD for real-time monitoring. The signals were recorded onto a micro SD memory card for offline processing and analysis. The purpose of the project was to have a better understanding of the wrist pulse wave signal and to assist the ayurvedic practitioner to detect pulse wave signal [90]. Clinicians today have limited examination of the pulse to its rate, rhythm, and volume by virtue of which they hardly come to a concrete diagnosis based upon pulse alone. If there could be a system by which the radial pulse could be critically examined just like the ancient ayurvedic practitioners and others, it could be one of the most useful tools in the field of noninvasive modern medical diagnosis of disease [136]. However, the relationship between radial pulse and cardiovascular disease is not well understood yet and leaves much space for further research. Modern medicine believes that a complete physical exam has always included observing palpation of arterial pulses; the intensity, rate, and rhythm and whether any blood vessel tenderness, tortuosity, or nodularity exists. These qualities can be seen using a noninvasive method only by an ECG signal. The radial artery pulse at the wrist is most commonly used and is adequate for assessing rate and rhythm, but it is not the best artery to indicate pulse character to do a complete physical exam [368]. Therefore, the radial signal obtained from the wrist is a harder method to examine the heart unless the noninvasive radial signal is converted to an invasive aortic signal. These aortic signals can be further analyzed and compared with cardiovascular model output aortic signals to have a better understanding of the blood flow in the cardiovascular circulatory system.

This overall review evoked the idea of using modern electronic sensors as a solution to obtain the wrist pulse signal of a patient more objectively. The wrist pulse signal can be collected using either a pressure sensor, photoelectric sensor, or ultrasonic sensor. These three sensors collect data noninvasively, which means there will be no puncturing of the skin, but instead, data can be collected by administering a wearable device with the sensor built into the patient. The wrist radial artery is the closest to the skin surface, making it easy to sense the changes in pressure noninvasively [87]. Thus, making devices such as watches and bracelets that can be worn around the wrist is the best choice of design for a wearable device. The wearable device can ensure continuous monitoring of the user's heart condition and indicate if there is any risk of circulatory blockage. By establishing a proper monitoring wearable device as stated in this review paper, this ideology will permit further work on other bloodstream interlinked diseases, such as pulmonary disease (respiratory failure, pulmonary edema, and so on), cerebrovascular disease (stroke), and so on because the organs in the human body are interlinked with the bloodstream. For instance, when a patient is having a respiratory issue, the blood flow from the lungs to the heart will be disrupted due to a shortage of oxygenated blood. This will give trouble to the heart to siphon blood to the systemic loop in the cardiovascular system. Thus, by using this philosophy, future studies can be carried out on other noncardiovascular diseases, which are interlinked with blood flow. Furthermore, there are a lot of emphasizing studies on central aortic blood pressure waveform as a better predictor of future cardiovascular diseases and all-cause mortality than peripheral blood pressure waveform [202, 203].

There is a lot of motivation in measuring central blood pressure noninvasively in the medical world [64]. Researchers are driven by the evidence that the central aortic blood pressure waveform provides a better assessment of cardiovascular risk [199, 369–372]. Upon a positive outcome from further studies, a wearable device shall be developed by converting radial blood pressure waveform to aortic blood pressure waveform to indicate the risk factors of the device's user towards having cardiovascular disease risk. Using the alerts from the device, the user can seek further consultation and the necessary medical treatment. In a nutshell, the proposed wearable device incorporating the abovementioned reviewed cardiovascular detection techniques shall enable its user to be well informed on his/her cardiovascular health risk.

References

[1] S. Kohno, A. L. Keenan, J. M. Ntambi, and M. Miyazaki, "Lipidomic insight into cardiovascular diseases," *Biochem. Biophys. Res. Commun.*, vol. 504, no. 3, pp. 590–595, Oct. 2018, doi: 10.1016/j.bbrc.2018.04.106

[2] I. Dadgar and T. Norström, "Is there a link between cardiovascular mortality and economic fluctuations?," *Scand. J. Public Health*, vol. 48, no. 7, 770–780, Jan. 2020, doi: 10.1177/1403494819890699

[3] D. Ramachandran, V. Ponnusamy Thangapandian, and H. Rajaguru, "Computerized approach for cardiovascular risk level detection using photoplethysmography signals," *Measurement*, vol. 150, 107048, Jan. 2020, doi: 10.1016/j.measurement.2019.107048

[4] W.-H. Lin, H. Zhang, and Y.-T. Zhang, "Investigation on cardiovascular risk prediction using physiological parameters," *Comput. Math. Methods Med.*, vol. 2013, pp. 1–21, 2013, doi: 10.1155/2013/272691

[5] S. M. Grundy et al., "Primary prevention of coronary heart disease: guidance from Framingham," *Circulation*, vol. 97, no. 18, pp. 1876–1887, May 1998, doi: 10.1161/01.CIR.97.18.1876

[6] J. R. Downs et al., "Primary prevention of acute coronary events with lovastatin in men and women with average cholesterol levels," *JAMA*, vol. 279, no. 20, p. 1615, May 1998, doi: 10.1001/jama.279.20.1615

[7] A. J. Alves et al., "Physical activity in primary and secondary prevention of cardiovascular disease: Overview updated," *World J. Cardiol.*, vol. 8, no. 10, p. 575, 2016, doi: 10.4330/wjc.v8.i10.575

[8] S. S. Gottlieb, R. J. McCarter, and R. A. Vogel, "Effect of beta-blockade on mortality among high-risk and low-risk patients after myocardial infarction," *Surv. Anesthesiol.*, vol. 43, no. 4, pp. 201–202, Aug. 1999, doi: 10.1097/00132586-199908000-00014

[9] Scandinavian Simvastatin Survival Study Group, "Randomised trial of cholesterol lowering in 4444 patients with coronary heart disease: the Scandinavian Simvastatin Survival Study (4S)," *Lancet*, vol. 344, no. 8934, Nov. 1994, doi: 10.1016/S0140-6736(94)90566-5

[10] The Long-Term Intervention with Pravastatin in Ischaemic Disease (LIPID) Study Group, "Prevention of cardiovascular events and death with pravastatin in patients with coronary heart disease and a broad range of initial cholesterol levels," *N. Engl. J. Med.*, vol. 339, no. 19, pp. 1349–1357, Nov. 1998, doi: 10.1056/NEJM199811053391902

[11] J. Wtorek, A. Bujnowski, J. Rumiński, A. Poliński, M. Kaczmarek, and A. Nowakowski, "Assessment of cardiovascular risk in assisted living," *Metrol. Meas. Syst.*, vol. 19, no. 2, pp. 231–244, Jan. 2012, doi: 10.2478/v10178-012-0020-0

[12] N. K. Wenger, "Cardiovascular disease in the elderly," *Cardiology*, vol. 74, no. 4, pp. 310–315, 1987, doi: 10.1159/000174216

[13] J. Allen, "Photoplethysmography and its application in clinical physiological measurement," *Physiol. Meas.*, vol. 28, no. 3, pp. R1–R39, Mar. 2007, doi: 10.1088/0967-3334/28/3/R01

[14] S. Xu et al., "Soft microfluidic assemblies of sensors, circuits, and radios for the skin," *Science*, vol. 344, no. 6179, pp. 70–74, Apr. 2014, doi: 10.1126/science.1250169

[15] S. Chen et al., "Hierarchical elastomer tuned self-powered pressure sensor for wearable multifunctional cardiovascular electronics," *Nano Energy*, vol. 70, 104460, Apr. 2020, doi: 10.1016/j.nanoen.2020.104460

[16] S. P. Karunathilake and G. U. Ganegoda, "Secondary prevention of cardiovascular diseases and application of technology for early diagnosis," *Biomed Res. Int.*, vol. 2018, pp. 1–9, 2018, doi: 10.1155/2018/5767864

[17] P. Brindle, A. Beswick, T. Fahey, and S. Ebrahim, "Accuracy and impact of risk assessment in the primary prevention of cardiovascular disease: a systematic review," *Heart*, vol. 92, no. 12, pp. 1752–1759, 2006, doi: 10.1136/hrt.2006.087932

[18] S. Patel, H. Park, P. Bonato, L. Chan, and M. Rodgers, "A review of wearable sensors and systems with application in rehabilitation," *J. Neuroengineering Rehabil.*, vol. 9, pp. 1–17, 2012. Available: https://jneuroengrehab.biomed central.com/articles/10.1186/1743-0003-9-21

[19] H. McGuire and B. H. Weigl, "Medical devices and diagnostics for cardiovascular diseases in low-resource settings," *J. Cardiovasc. Transl. Res.*, vol. 7, no. 8, pp. 737–748, 2014, doi: 10.1007/s12265-014-9591-3

[20] P. Roriz, O. Frazão, A. B. Lobo-Ribeiro, J. L. Santos, and J. A. Simões, "Review of fiber-optic pressure sensors for biomedical and biomechanical applications," *J. Biomed. Opt.*, vol. 18, no. 5, 050903, 2013, doi: 10.1117/1.jbo.18.5.050903

[21] T. G. Stavropoulos, A. Papastergiou, L. Mpaltadoros, S. Nikolopoulos, and I. Kompatsiaris, "IoT wearable sensors and devices in elderly care: A literature review," *Sensors (Switzerland)*, vol. 20, no. 10, 2020, doi: 10.3390/s20102826

[22] G. E. MacKinnon and E. L. Brittain, "Mobile health technologies in cardiopulmonary disease," *Chest*, vol. 157, no. 3, pp. 654–664, 2020, doi: 10.1016/j.chest.2019.10.015

[23] Z. Altintas, W. M. Fakanya, and I. E. Tothill, "Cardiovascular disease detection using bio-sensing techniques," *Talanta*, vol. 128, pp. 177–186, 2014, doi: 10.1016/j.talanta.2014.04.060

[24] A. R. Castro, S. O. Silva, and S. C. Soares, "The use of high sensitivity C-reactive protein in cardiovascular disease detection," *J. Pharm. Pharm. Sci.*, vol. 21, pp. 496–503, Nov. 2018, doi: 10.18433/jpps29872

[25] J. H. Park, D. Dehaini, J. Zhou, M. Holay, R. H. Fang, and L. Zhang, "Biomimetic nanoparticle technology for cardiovascular disease detection and treatment," *Nanoscale Horizons*, vol. 5, no. 1, pp. 25–42, 2020, doi: 10.1039/c9nh00291j

[26] Y. Shi, P. Lawford, and R. Hose, "Review of zero-D and 1-D models of blood flow in the cardiovascular system," *Biomed. Eng. Online*, vol. 10, no. 1, p. 33, 2011, doi: 10.1186/1475-925X-10-33

[27] P. Reymond, O. Vardoulis, and N. Stergiopulos, "Generic and patient-specific models of the arterial tree," *J. Clin. Monit. Comput.*, vol. 26, no. 5, pp. 375–382, 2012, doi: 10.1007/s10877-012-9382-9

[28] A. D. McCulloch, "Systems biophysics: Multiscale biophysical modeling of organ systems," *Biophys. J.*, vol. 110, no. 5, pp. 1023–1027, 2016, doi: 10.1016/j.bpj.2016.02.007

[29] E. Fatahian, N. Kordani, and H. Fatahian, "The application of computational fluid dynamics (CFD) method and several rheological models of blood flow: A review," *Gazi Univ. J. Sci.*, vol. 31, no. 4, pp. 1213–1227, 2018.

[30] P. G. Morton, "Anatomy and physiology of the cardiovascular system," *Crit. Care Nurs. A Holist. Approach*, pp. 193–205, 2013, doi: 10.1016/s1089-9472(97)80029-9

[31] H. A. L. Mossa, "Engineering modeling of human cardiovascular system," *NJES*, vol. 1111, no. 22, pp. 307–314, 2008.

[32] H. Mohammadi and K. Mequanint, "Prosthetic aortic heart valves: Modeling and design," *Med. Eng. Phys.*, vol. 33, no. 2, pp. 131–147, 2011, doi: 10.1016/j.medengphy.2010.09.017. https://tinylink.info/10cuq

[33] K. Moore, A. Dalley, and A. Agur, *Clinically Oriented*, 1999. Lippincott Williams & Wilkins.

[34] P. I. Aaronson, J. P. T. Ward, and M. J. Connolly, *"The circulatory system,"* 2009, pp. 471–522.

[35] European Environment Agency (EEA). *"Cardiovascular physiology concepts, second edition,"* vol. 53, no. 9. 2019.

[36] D. Mozaffarian et al., "Executive summary: Heart disease and stroke statistics—2015 update," *Circulation*, vol. 131, no. 4, pp. 434–441, Jan. 2015, doi: 10.1161/CIR.0000000000000157

[37] M. Nichols, N. Townsend, P. Scarborough, and M. Rayner, "Cardiovascular disease in Europe 2014: Epidemiological update," *Eur. Heart J.*, vol. 35, no. 42, pp. 2950–2959, 2014, doi: 10.1093/eurheartj/ehu299

[38] O. Faust, U. R. Acharya, F. Molinari, S. Chattopadhyay, and T. Tamura, "Linear and non-linear analysis of cardiac health in diabetic subjects," *Biomed. Signal Process. Control*, vol. 7, no. 3, pp. 295–302, May 2012, doi: 10.1016/j.bspc.2011.06.002

[39] G. A. Mensah and D. W. Brown, "An overview of cardiovascular disease burden in The United States," *Health Aff.*, vol. 26, no. 1, pp. 38–48, Jan. 2007, doi: 10.1377/hlthaff.26.1.38

[40] R. Ross, "The pathogenesis of atherosclerosis—An update," *N. Engl. J. Med.*, vol. 314, no. 8, pp. 488–500, Feb. 1986, doi: 10.1056/NEJM198602203140806

[41] D. G. Hackam and S. S. Anand, "Emerging risk factors for atherosclerotic vascular disease," *JAMA*, vol. 290, no. 7, p. 932, Aug. 2003, doi: 10.1001/jama.290.7.932

[42] R. A. Vogel, "Coronary risk factors, endothelial function, and atherosclerosis: A review," *Clin. Cardiol.*, vol. 20, no. 5, pp. 426–432, May 1997, doi: 10.1002/clc.4960200505

[43]   D. H. O'Leary, J. F. Polak, R. A. Kronmal, T. A. Manolio, G. L. Burke, and S. K. Wolfson, "Carotid-artery intima and media thickness as a risk factor for myocardial infarction and stroke in older adults," *N. Engl. J. Med.*, vol. 340, no. 1, pp. 14–22, Jan. 1999, doi: 10.1056/NEJM199901073400103

[44]   P. Amarenco et al., "Atherosclerotic disease of the aortic arch and the risk of ischemic stroke," *N. Engl. J. Med.*, vol. 331, no. 22, pp. 1474–1479, Dec. 1994, doi: 10.1056/NEJM199412013312202

[45]   G. De Luca, H. Suryapranata, J. P. Ottervanger, and E. M. Antman, "Time delay to treatment and mortality in primary angioplasty for acute myocardial infarction," *Circulation*, vol. 109, no. 10, pp. 1223–1225, Mar. 2004, doi: 10.1161/01.CIR.0000121424.76486.20

[46]   F. L. Silver, J. W. Norris, A. J. Lewis, and V. C. Hachinski, "Early mortality following stroke: a prospective review," *Stroke*, vol. 15, no. 3, pp. 492–496, May 1984, doi: 10.1161/01.STR.15.3.492

[47]   H. A. L. Mossa, "Engineering modeling of human cardiovascular system," in S. M. Becker and A. V. Kuznetsov (eds), *Modeling of Microscale Transport in Biological Processes*, pp. 147–161. Springer.

[48]   J. Stewart, G. Manmathan, and P. Wilkinson, "Primary prevention of cardiovascular disease: A review of contemporary guidance and literature," *JRSM Cardiovasc. Dis.*, vol. 6, 204800401668721, Jan. 2017, doi: 10.1177/2048004016687211

[49]   T. A. Pearson et al., "AHA guidelines for primary prevention of cardiovascular disease and stroke: 2002 Update," *Circulation*, vol. 106, no. 3, pp. 388–391, Jul. 2002, doi: 10.1161/01.CIR.0000020190.45892.75

[50]   E. Archer and S. N. Blair, "Physical activity and the prevention of cardiovascular disease: from evolution to epidemiology," *Prog. Cardiovasc. Dis.*, vol. 53, no. 6, pp. 387–396, May 2011, doi: 10.1016/j.pcad.2011.02.006

[51]   J. H. Park, D. Dehaini, J. Zhou, M. Holay, R. H. Fang, and L. Zhang, "Biomimetic nanoparticle technology for cardiovascular disease detection and treatment," *Nanoscale Horiz.*, vol. 5, no. 1, pp. 25–42, 2020, doi: 10.1039/C9NH00291J

[52]   J. Sanz and Z. A. Fayad, "Imaging of atherosclerotic cardiovascular disease," *Nature*, vol. 451, no. 7181, pp. 953–957, Feb. 2008, doi: 10.1038/nature06803

[53]   D. S. Celermajer, C. K. Chow, E. Marijon, N. M. Anstey, and K. S. Woo, "Cardiovascular disease in the developing world," *J. Am. Coll. Cardiol.*, vol. 60, no. 14, pp. 1207–1216, Oct. 2012, doi: 10.1016/j.jacc.2012.03.074

[54]   H. Clark, "NCDs: a challenge to sustainable human development," *Lancet*, vol. 381, no. 9866, pp. 510–511, Feb. 2013, doi: 10.1016/S0140-6736(13)60058-6

[55]   G. A. Roth et al., "Global, regional, and national burden of cardiovascular diseases for 10 causes, 1990 to 2015," *J. Am. Coll. Cardiol.*, vol. 70, no. 1, pp. 1–25, Jul. 2017, doi: 10.1016/j.jacc.2017.04.052

[56]   X. Yan, L. Zhang, J. Li, D. Du, and F. Hou, "Entropy-based measures of hypnopompic heart rate variability contribute to the automatic prediction of cardiovascular events," *Entropy*, vol. 22, no. 2, p. 241, Feb. 2020, doi: 10.3390/e22020241

[57]   R. Manfredini et al., "Twenty-four-hour patterns in occurrence and pathophysiology of acute cardiovascular events and ischemic heart disease,"

Chronobiol. Int., vol. 30, no. 1–2, pp. 6–16, Mar. 2013, doi: 10.3109/07420528.2012.715843

[58] E. A. Goff, C. L. Nicholas, A. K. Simonds, J. Trinder, and M. J. Morrell, "Differential effects of waking from non-rapid eye movement versus rapid eye movement sleep on cardiovascular activity," *J. Sleep Res.*, vol. 19, no. 1p2, pp. 201–206, Mar. 2010, doi: 10.1111/j.1365-2869.2009.00783.x

[59] Q. Wang, Y. Cui, P. Yogendranath, and N. Wang, "Blood pressure and heart rate variability are linked with hyperphosphatemia in chronic kidney disease patients," *Chronobiol. Int.*, vol. 35, no. 10, pp. 1329–1334, Oct. 2018, doi: 10.1080/07420528.2018.1486850

[60] N. Takeda and K. Maemura, "Circadian clock and the onset of cardiovascular events," *Hypertens. Res.*, vol. 39, no. 6, pp. 383–390, Jun. 2016, doi: 10.1038/hr.2016.9

[61] A. Amici et al., "Exaggerated morning blood pressure surge and cardiovascular events. A 5-year longitudinal study in normotensive and well-controlled hypertensive elderly," *Arch. Gerontol. Geriatr.*, vol. 49, no. 2, pp. e105–e109, Sep. 2009, doi: 10.1016/j.archger.2008.10.003

[62] R. Furlan et al., "Continuous 24-hour assessment of the neural regulation of systemic arterial pressure and RR variabilities in ambulant subjects," *Circulation*, vol. 81, no. 2, pp. 537–547, Feb. 1990, doi: 10.1161/01.CIR.81.2.537

[63] P. Van de Borne, H. Nguyen, P. Biston, P. Linkowski, and J. P. Degaute, "Effects of wake and sleep stages on the 24-h autonomic control of blood pressure and heart rate in recumbent men," *Am. J. Physiol. Circ. Physiol.*, vol. 266, no. 2, pp. H548–H554, Feb. 1994, doi: 10.1152/ajpheart.1994.266.2.H548

[64] E. Agabiti-Rosei et al., "Central blood pressure measurements and antihypertensive therapy: A consensus document," *Hypertension*, vol. 50, no. 1, pp. 154–160, 2007, doi: 10.1161/HYPERTENSIONAHA.107.090068

[65] G. Mancia, "Effects of blood-pressure measurement by the doctor on patient's blood pressure and heart rate," *Lancet*, vol. 322, no. 8352, pp. 695–698, Sep. 1983, doi: 10.1016/S0140-6736(83)92244-4

[66] P. Pickering, "Blood pressure measurement and detection of hypertension," *Lancet*, vol. 344, no. 8914, pp. 31–35, Jul. 1994, doi: 10.1016/S0140-6736(94)91053-7

[67] M. L. Aisen, H. I. Krebs, N. Hogan, F. McDowell, and B. T. Volpe, "The effect of robot-assisted therapy and rehabilitative training on motor recovery following stroke," *Arch. Neurol.*, vol. 54, no. 4, pp. 443–446, Apr. 1997, doi: 10.1001/archneur.1997.00550160075019

[68] E. A. Crisostomo, P. W. Duncan, M. Propst, D. V. Dawson, and J. N. Davis, "Evidence that amphetamine with physical therapy promotes recovery of motor function in stroke patients," *Ann. Neurol.*, vol. 23, no. 1, pp. 94–97, Jan. 1988, doi: 10.1002/ana.410230117

[69] H. Thomas et al., "Global atlas of cardiovascular disease 2000-2016: the path to prevention and control," *Glob. Heart*, vol. 13, no. 3, pp. 143–163, 2018, doi: 10.1016/j.gheart.2018.09.511

[70] GBD 2013 Mortality and Causes of Death Collaborators, "Global, regional, and national age–sex specific all-cause and cause-specific mortality for 240

causes of death, 1990–2013: a systematic analysis for the Global Burden of Disease Study 2013," *Lancet*, vol. 385, no. 9963, pp. 117–171, Jan. 2015, doi: 10.1016/S0140-6736(14)61682-2

[71] D. M. Lloyd-Jones et al., "Parental cardiovascular disease as a risk factor for cardiovascular disease in middle-aged adults," *JAMA*, vol. 291, no. 18, 2204, May 2004, doi: 10.1001/jama.291.18.2204

[72] J. A. Finegold, P. Asaria, and D. P. Francis, "Mortality from ischaemic heart disease by country, region, and age: Statistics from World Health Organisation and United Nations," *Int. J. Cardiol.*, vol. 168, no. 2, pp. 934–945, Sep. 2013, doi: 10.1016/j.ijcard.2012.10.046

[73] A. H. E. M. Maas and Y. E. A. Appelman, "Gender differences in coronary heart disease," *Neth. Hear. J.*, vol. 18, no. 12, pp. 598–603, Nov. 2010, doi: 10.1007/s12471-010-0841-y

[74] P. Jousilahti, E. Vartiainen, J. Tuomilehto, and P. Puska, "Sex, age, cardio-vascular risk factors, and coronary heart disease," *Circulation*, vol. 99, no. 9, pp. 1165–1172, Mar. 1999, doi: 10.1161/01.CIR.99.9.1165

[75] T. A. Gaziano, A. Bitton, S. Anand, S. Abrahams-Gessel, and A. Murphy, "Growing epidemic of coronary heart disease in low- and middle-income countries," *Curr. Probl. Cardiol.*, vol. 35, no. 2, pp. 72–115, Feb. 2010, doi: 10.1016/j.cpcardiol.2009.10.002

[76] M. E. Safar, B. I. Levy, and H. Struijker-Boudier, "Current perspectives on arterial stiffness and pulse pressure in hypertension and cardiovascular diseases," *Circulation*, vol. 107, no. 22, pp. 2864–2869, 2003, doi: 10.1161/01.CIR.0000069826.36125.B4

[77] J. E. Hall and A. C. Guyton. *Guyton and Hall Textbook of Medical Physiology*. Elsevier.

[78] T. Pereira, C. Correia, and J. Cardoso, "Novel methods for pulse wave velocity measurement," *J. Med. Biol. Eng.*, vol. 35, no. 5, pp. 555–565, 2015, doi: 10.1007/s40846-015-0086-8

[79] V. Krasteva, I. Jekova, R. Leber, R. Schmid, and R. Abächerli, "Real-time arrhythmia detection with supplementary ECG quality and pulse wave monitoring for the reduction of false alarms in ICUs," *Physiol. Meas.*, vol. 37, no. 8, pp. 1273–1297, Aug. 2016, doi: 10.1088/0967-3334/37/8/1273

[80] W. Ping, W. Jin-gang, S. Xiao-bo, and H. Wei, "The research of telemedicine system based on embedded computer," *Conf. Proc. IEEE Eng. Med. Biol. Soc.*, vol. 25, no. 6, pp. 114–117, 2005, doi: 10.1109/IEMBS.2005.1616355

[81] H. S. Ng, M. L. Sim, C. M. Tan, and C. C. Wong, "Wireless technologies for telemedicine," *BT Technol. J.*, vol. 24, no. 2, pp. 130–137, Apr. 2006, doi: 10.1007/s10550-006-0050-9

[82] A. M. Johansson, I. Lindberg, and S. Söderberg, "Patients' experiences with specialist care via video consultation in primary healthcare in rural areas," *Int. J. Telemed. Appl.*, vol. 2014, pp. 1–7, 2014, doi: 10.1155/2014/143824

[83] P. Kakria, N. K. Tripathi, and P. Kitipawang, "A real-time health monitoring system for remote cardiac patients using smartphone and wearable sensors," *Int. J. Telemed. Appl.*, vol. 2015, 2015, doi: 10.1155/2015/373474

[84] L. Ricciardi, F. Mostashari, J. Murphy, J. G. Daniel, and E. P. Siminerio, "A National action plan to support consumer engagement via E-health," *Health Aff.*, vol. 32, no. 2, pp. 376–384, Feb. 2013, doi: 10.1377/hlthaff.2012.1216

[85] R. Say, M. Murtagh, and R. Thomson, "Patients' preference for involvement in medical decision making: A narrative review," *Patient Educ. Couns.*, vol. 60, no. 2, pp. 102–114, Feb. 2006, doi: 10.1016/j.pec.2005.02.003

[86] X. Chen, C. T. Ho, E. T. Lim, and T. Z. Kyaw, "Cellular phone based online ECG processing for ambulatory and continuous detection," *Comput. Cardiol.*, Sep. 2007, pp. 653–656, doi: 10.1109/CIC.2007.4745570

[87] K. W. Goh, J. Lavanya, E. K. Tan, C. B. Soh, and Y. Kim, "A PDA-based ECG beat detector for home cardiac care," in *2005 IEEE Engineering in Medicine and Biology 27th Annual Conference*, 2005, pp. 375–378, doi: 10.1109/IEMBS.2005.1616423

[88] J. Rodriguez, A. Goni, and A. Illarramendi, "Real-time classification of ECGs on a PDA," *IEEE Trans. Inf. Technol. Biomed.*, vol. 9, no. 1, pp. 23–34, Mar. 2005, doi: 10.1109/TITB.2004.838369

[89] Z. Jin, Y. Sun, and A. C. Cheng, "Predicting cardiovascular disease from real-time electrocardiographic monitoring: An adaptive machine learning approach on a cell phone," in *2009 Annual International Conference of the IEEE Engineering in Medicine and Biology Society*, Sep. 2009, pp. 6889–6892, doi: 10.1109/IEMBS.2009.5333610

[90] J. J. Oresko et al., "A wearable smartphone-based platform for real-time cardiovascular disease detection via electrocardiogram processing," *IEEE Trans. Inf. Technol. Biomed.*, vol. 14, no. 3, pp. 734–740, 2010, doi: 10.1109/TITB.2010.2047865

[91] J. M. Cano-Garcia, E. Gonzalez-Parada, V. Alarcon-Collantes, and E. Casilari-Perez., "A PDA-based portable wireless ECG monitor for medical personal area networks," in *MELECON 2006–2006 IEEE Mediterranean Electrotechnical Conference*, 2006, pp. 713–716, doi: 10.1109/MELCON.2006.1653199

[92] W.-Y. Chung, C.-L. Yau, K.-S. Shin, and R. Myllyla, "A cell phone based health monitoring system with self analysis processor using wireless sensor network technology," in *2007 29th Annual International Conference of the IEEE Engineering in Medicine and Biology Society*, Aug. 2007, pp. 3705–3708, doi: 10.1109/IEMBS.2007.4353136

[93] T.-S. Lee, J.-H. Hong, and M.-C. Cho, "Biomedical digital assistant for ubiquitous healthcare," in *2007 29th Annual International Conference of the IEEE Engineering in Medicine and Biology Society*, Aug. 2007, pp. 1790–1793, doi: 10.1109/IEMBS.2007.4352659

[94] G. Appelboom et al., "Smart wearable body sensors for patient self-assessment and monitoring," *Arch. public Heal.*, vol. 72, no. 1, p. 28, 2014, doi: 10.1186/2049-3258-72-28

[95] P. Bonato, "Advances in wearable technology and applications in physical medicine and rehabilitation," *J. Neuroeng. Rehabil.*, vol. 2, p. 2, 2005, doi: 10.1186/1743-0003-2-2

[96] S. Meystre, "The current state of telemonitoring: A comment on the literature," *Telemed. e-Health*, vol. 11, no. 1, pp. 63–69, Feb. 2005, doi: 10.1089/tmj.2005.11.63

[97] K. Hung, Y. T. Zhang, and B. Tai, "Wearable medical devices for tele-home healthcare," in *The 26th Annual International Conference of the IEEE Engineering in Medicine and Biology Society*, vol. 4, pp. 5384–5387, doi: 10.1109/IEMBS.2004.1404503

[98] D. Phan, L. Y. Siong, P. N. Pathirana, and A. Seneviratne, "Smartwatch: Performance evaluation for long-term heart rate monitoring," in *2015 International Symposium on Bioelectronics and Bioinformatics (ISBB)*, Oct. 2015, pp. 144–147, doi: 10.1109/ISBB.2015.7344944

[99] F. Jing et al., "The influence on medical activities by mobile medical application," in *2018 4th Annual International Conference on Network and Information Systems for Computers (ICNISC)*, Apr. 2018, pp. 104–106, doi: 10.1109/ICNISC.2018.00028

[100] P. Athilingam, M. A. Labrador, E. F. J. Remo, L. Mack, A. B. San Juan, and A. F. Elliott, "Features and usability assessment of a patient-centered mobile application (HeartMapp) for self-management of heart failure," *Appl. Nurs. Res.*, vol. 32, pp. 156–163, Nov. 2016, doi: 10.1016/j.apnr.2016.07.001

[101] B. H. Dobkin and A. Dorsch, "The Promise of mHealth," *Neurorehabil. Neural Repair*, vol. 25, no. 9, pp. 788–798, Nov. 2011, doi: 10.1177/1545968311425908

[102] A. Darwish and A. E. Hassanien, "Wearable and implantable wireless sensor network solutions for healthcare monitoring," *Sensors*, vol. 11, no. 6, pp. 5561–5595, May 2011, doi: 10.3390/s110605561

[103] S. Wassertheurer et al., "A new oscillometric method for pulse wave analysis: Comparison with a common tonometric method," *J. Hum. Hypertens.*, vol. 24, no. 8, pp. 498–504, 2010, doi: 10.1038/jhh.2010.27

[104] I. G. Horváth et al., "Invasive validation of a new oscillometric device (Arteriograph) for measuring augmentation index, central blood pressure and aortic pulse wave velocity," *J. Hypertens.*, vol. 28, no. 10, 2010. Available: https://journals.lww.com/jhypertension/Fulltext/2010/10000/Invasive_validation_of_a_new_oscillometric_device.15.aspx

[105] N. B. Rossen et al., "Invasive validation of arteriograph estimates of central blood pressure in patients with type 2 diabetes," *Am. J. Hypertens.*, vol. 27, no. 5, pp. 674–679, 2014, doi: 10.1093/ajh/hpt162

[106] A. Lowe, W. Harrison, E. El-Aklouk, P. Ruygrok, and A. M. Al-Jumaily, "Non-invasive model-based estimation of aortic pulse pressure using suprasystolic brachial pressure waveforms," *J. Biomech.*, vol. 42, no. 13, pp. 2111–2115, 2009, doi: 10.1016/j.jbiomech.2009.05.029

[107] S. A. Koudryavtcev and V. M. Lazarev, "Validation of the BPLab® 24-hour blood pressure monitoring system according to the European standard BS EN 1060-4:2004 and British Hypertension Society protocol," *Med. Devices Evid. Res.*, vol. 4, no. 1, pp. 193–196, 2011, doi: 10.2147/MDER.S25800

[108] C. Ott, S. Haetinger, M. P. Schneider, M. Pauschinger, and R. E. Schmieder, "Comparison of two noninvasive devices for measurement of central

systolic blood pressure with invasive measurement during cardiac catheterization," *J. Clin. Hypertens.*, vol. 14, no. 9, pp. 575–579, 2012, doi: 10.1111/j.1751-7176.2012.00682.x

[109] B. Williams, P. S. Lacy, P. Yan, C.-N. Hwee, C. Liang, and C.-M. Ting, "Development and validation of a novel method to derive central aortic systolic pressure from the radial pressure waveform using an N-point moving average method," *J. Am. Coll. Cardiol.*, vol. 57, no. 8, pp. 951–961, Feb. 2011, doi: 10.1016/j.jacc.2010.09.054

[110] B. Williams, P. S. Lacy, F. Baschiera, P. Brunel, and R. Düsing, "Novel description of the 24-hour circadian rhythms of brachial versus central aortic blood pressure and the impact of blood pressure treatment in a randomized controlled clinical trial: The ambulatory central aortic pressure (AMCAP) study," *Hypertension*, vol. 61, no. 6, pp. 1168–1176, 2013, doi: 10.1161/HYPERTENSIONAHA.111.00763

[111] S. E. Brett, A. Guilcher, B. Clapp, and P. Chowienczyk, "Estimating central systolic blood pressure during oscillometric determination of blood pressure: Proof of concept and validation by comparison with intra-aortic pressure recording and arterial tonometry," *Blood Press. Monit.*, vol. 17, no. 3, 2012. Available: https://journals.lww.com/bpmonitoring/Fulltext/2012/06000/Estimating_central_systolic_blood_pressure_during.8.aspx

[112] T. Pereira et al., "Invasive validation of the Complior Analyse in the assessment of central artery pressure curves: a methodological study," *Blood Press. Monit.*, vol. 19, no. 5, 2014. Available: https://journals.lww.com/bpmonitoring/Fulltext/2014/10000/Invasive_validation_of_the_Complior_Analyse_in_the.6.aspx

[113] S.-S. Chio, *"Pulse dynamics. non-invasive blood pressure and hemodynamic monitoring,"* vol. 2013, pp. 0–146, March 2002.

[114] P. Salvi, "Is validation of non-invasive hemodynamic measurement devices actually required?," *Hypertens. Res.*, vol. 37, no. 1, pp. 7–9, 2014, doi: 10.1038/hr.2013.115

[115] G. Swamy, D. Xu, N. B. Olivier, and R. Mukkamala, "An adaptive transfer function for deriving the aortic pressure waveform from a peripheral artery pressure waveform," *Am. J. Physiol. Hear. Circ. Physiol.*, vol. 297, no. 5, pp. 1956–1963, 2009, doi: 10.1152/ajpheart.00155.2009

[116] K. Takazawa, H. Kobayashi, N. Shindo, N. Tanaka, and A. Yamashina, "Relationship between radial and central aeterial pulse wave and evaluation of central aortic pressure using the radial arterial pulse wave," *Hypertens. Res.*, vol. 30, no. 3, pp. 219–228, 2007, doi: 10.1291/hypres.30.219

[117] K. Takazawa et al., "Estimation of central aortic systolic pressure using late systolic inflection of radial artery pulse and its application to vasodilator therapy," *J. Hypertens.*, vol. 30, no. 5, 2012. Available: https://journals.lww.com/jhypertension/Fulltext/2012/05000/Estimation_of_central_aortic_systolic_pressure.14.aspx

[118] S. S. Hickson et al., "The accuracy of central SBP determined from the second systolic peak of the peripheral pressure waveform," *J. Hypertens.*, vol. 27, no. 9, 2009. Available: https://journals.lww.com/jhypertension/Fulltext/2009/09000/The_accuracy_of_central_SBP_determined_from_the.10.aspx

[119] F.-H. Ding, Y. Li, R.-Y. Zhang, Q. Zhang, and J.-G. Wang, "Comparison of the SphygmoCor and Omron devices in the estimation of pressure amplification against the invasive catheter measurement," *J. Hypertens.*, vol. 31, no. 1, 2013. Available: https://journals.lww.com/jhypertension/Fulltext/2013/01000/Comparison_of_the_SphygmoCor_and_Omron_devices_in.15.aspx

[120] T. Weber et al., "Validation of a brachial cuff-based method for estimating central systolic blood pressure," *Hypertension*, vol. 58, no. 5, pp. 825–832, 2011, doi: 10.1161/HYPERTENSIONAHA.111.176313

[121] R. Kelly and D. Fitchett, "Noninvasive determination of aortic input impedance and external left ventricular power output: A validation and repeatability study of a new technique," *J. Am. Coll. Cardiol.*, vol. 20, no. 4, pp. 952 LP – 963, Oct. 1992, doi: 10.1016/0735-1097(92)90198-V

[122] M. J. Burns, J. D. Seed, A. V. Incognito, C. J. Doherty, K. Notay, and P. J. Millar, "Comparison of laboratory and ambulatory measures of central blood pressure and pulse wave reflection: hitting the target or missing the mark?," *J. Am. Soc. Hypertens.*, vol. 12, no. 4, pp. 275–284, Apr. 2018, doi: 10.1016/j.jash.2018.01.014

[123] P. Salvi, G. Lio, C. Labat, E. Ricci, B. Pannier, and A. Benetos, "Validation of a new non-invasive portable tonometer for determining arterial pressure wave and pulse wave velocity: the PulsePen device," *J. Hypertens.*, vol. 22, no. 12, 2004. Available: https://journals.lww.com/jhypertension/Fulltext/2004/12000/Validation_of_a_new_non_invasive_portable.10.aspx

[124] Y. Yao, L. Wang, L. Hao, L. Xu, S. Zhou, and W. Liu, "The noninvasive measurement of central aortic blood pressure waveform," in *Blood Pressure – from Bench to Bed*, 2018. InTechOpen. 10.5772/intechopen.81335

[125] C.-H. Chen et al., "Estimation of central aortic pressure waveform by mathematical transformation of radial tonometry pressure," *Circulation*, vol. 95, no. 7, pp. 1827–1836, Apr. 1997, doi: 10.1161/01.CIR.95.7.1827

[126] A. L. Pauca, M. F. O'Rourke, and N. D. Kon, "Prospective evaluation of a method for estimating ascending aortic pressure from the radial artery pressure waveform," *Hypertension*, vol. 38, no. 4, pp. 932–937, 2001, doi: 10.1161/hy1001.096106

[127] G. Pucci et al., "Evaluation of the Vicorder, a novel cuff-based device for the noninvasive estimation of central blood pressure," *J. Hypertens.*, vol. 31, no. 1, pp. 77–85, Jan. 2013, doi: 10.1097/HJH.0b013e32835a8eb1

[128] H. Smulyan, D. S. Siddiqui, R. J. Carlson, G. M. London, and M. E. Safar, "Clinical utility of aortic pulses and pressures calculated from applanated radial-artery pulses," *Hypertension*, vol. 42, no. 2, pp. 150–155, 2003, doi: 10.1161/01.HYP.0000084051.34269.A9

[129] E. Laugesen et al., "Assessment of central blood pressure in patients with type 2 diabetes: A comparison between sphygmocor and invasively measured values," *Am. J. Hypertens.*, vol. 27, no. 2, pp. 169–176, 2014, doi: 10.1093/ajh/hpt195

[130] J. E. Sharman et al., "Validation of a generalized transfer function to noninvasively derive central blood pressure during exercise," *Hypertension*, vol. 47, no. 6, pp. 1203–1208, 2006, doi: 10.1161/01.HYP.0000223013.60612.72

[131] G. Pucci et al., "Validation of Vicorder & Sphygmocor with invasive blood pressure: PP.10.395," *J. Hypertens.*, vol. 28, p. S485, 2010. Available: https://journals.lww.com/jhypertension/Fulltext/2010/06001/VALIDATION_OF_VICORDER___SPHYGMOCOR_WITH_INVASIVE.485.aspx

[132] H. M. Cheng, S. H. Sung, Y. T. Shih, S. Y. Chuang, W. C. Yu, and C. H. Chen, "Measurement accuracy of a stand-alone oscillometric central blood pressure monitor: A validation report for microlife WatchBP office central," *Am. J. Hypertens.*, vol. 26, no. 1, pp. 42–50, 2013, doi: 10.1093/ajh/hps021

[133] Y. T. Shih, H. M. Cheng, S. H. Sung, W. C. Hu, and C. H. Chen, "Quantification of the calibration error in the transfer function-derived central aortic blood pressures," *Am. J. Hypertens.*, vol. 24, no. 12, pp. 1312–1317, 2011, doi: 10.1038/ajh.2011.146

[134] H. Nakano et al., "Self-monitoring of ambulatory blood pressure by the Microlife WatchBP O3--An application test," *Clin. Exp. Hypertens.*, vol. 33, no. 1, pp. 34–40, 2011, doi: 10.3109/10641963.2010.503300

[135] W. Zuo, P. Wang, and D. Zhang, "Comparison of three different types of wrist pulse signals by their physical meanings and diagnosis performance," *IEEE J. Biomed. Heal. Informatics*, vol. 20, no. 1, pp. 119–127, 2016, doi: 10.1109/JBHI.2014.2369821

[136] M. Sharmila Begum, R. Duraiarasan, and P. J. Dhivaakar, "Diagnosing diseases through pulse using pressure sensor," in *Proceedings – 2012 International Conference on Data Science & Engineering* 2012, no. July 2012, pp. 140–143, 2012, doi: 10.1109/ICDSE.2012.6281895

[137] Gösele, A. Heuberger, and H. Sandmaier, "A silicon capacitive absolute pressure sensor with programmable on-chip electronics," *Sens Actuators A: Phys.*, vol. 66, no. 1–3, pp. 207–212, 1998, doi: 10.1016/S0924-4247(98)00214-3

[138] S. Thakkar, "Wrist pulse acquisition and recording system," *Commun. Appl. Electron.*, vol. 1, no. 6, pp. 20–24, 2015.

[139] G. Schwartz et al., "Flexible polymer transistors with high pressure sensitivity for application in electronic skin and health monitoring," *Nat. Commun.*, vol. 4, no. 1, p. 1859, Oct. 2013, doi: 10.1038/ncomms2832

[140] "BPro 24 hour Smart Watch ABPM Blood Pressure Monitor, MedTach Canada," *MedTach*, 2019. www.bpro.ie (accessed Dec. 29, 2019).

[141] K-G. Ng, C-M. Ting, J-H. Yeo, K-W. Sim, W-L. Peh, N-H. Chua, N-K. Chua, and F. Kwong, "Progress on the development of the MediWatch ambulatory blood pressure monitor and related devices," *Blood Press. Monit.*, vol. 9, no. 3, pp. 149–165, 2004 *"Method and device for monitoring blood pressure,"* 2002, doi: 10.1097/01.mbp.0000130432.57658.f7

[142] H. Demirezen and C. E. Erdem, "An overview of non-contact photoplethysmography," *IEEE Proc.*, pp. 1–4, 2017, doi: 10.1109/siu.2017.7960176

[143] C. Fischer, B. Domer, T. Wibmer, and T. Penzel, "An algorithm for real-time pulse waveform segmentation and artifact detection in photoplethysmograms," *IEEE J. Biomed. Heal. Informatics*, vol. 21, no. 2, pp. 372–381, 2017, doi: 10.1109/JBHI.2016.2518202

[144] P. H. Lai and I. Kim, "Lightweight wrist photoplethysmography for heavy exercise: Motion robust heart rate monitoring algorithm," *Healthc. Technol. Lett.*, vol. 2, no. 1, pp. 6–11, 2015, doi: 10.1049/htl.2014.0097

[145] J. Spigulis, L. Gailite, A. Lihachev, and R. Erts, "Simultaneous recording of skin blood pulsations at different vascular depths by multiwavelength photoplethysmography," *Appl. Opt.*, vol. 46, no. 10, 1754, Apr. 2007, doi: 10.1364/AO.46.001754

[146] C. Wang et al., "Monitoring of the central blood pressure waveform via a conformal ultrasonic device," *Nat. Biomed. Eng.*, vol. 2, no. 9, pp. 687–695, 2018, doi: 10.1038/s41551-018-0287-x

[147] D. W. Holdsworth, C. J. D. Norley, R. Frayne, D. A. Steinman, and B. K. Rutt, "Characterization of common carotid artery blood-flow waveforms in normal human subjects," *Physiol. Meas.*, vol. 20, no. 3, pp. 219–240, Aug. 1999, doi: 10.1088/0967-3334/20/3/301

[148] L. Jonveaux, "Arduino-like development kit for single-element ultrasound imaging," *J. Open Hardw.*, vol. 1, no. 1, 2017, doi: 10.5334/joh.2

[149] C. Yapijakis, "Hippocrates of Kos, the father of clinical medicine, and asclepiades of Bithynia, the father of molecular medicine," *In Vivo*, vol. 23, no. 4, pp. 507–514, 2009.

[150] S.-C. Cheng et al., "Fire-heat and Qi deficiency syndromes as predictors of short-term prognosis of acute ischemic stroke," *J. Altern. Complement. Med.*, vol. 19, no. 8, pp. 721–728, Aug. 2013, doi: 10.1089/acm.2012.0546

[151] J. Xu and Y. Yang, "Traditional Chinese medicine in the Chinese health care system," *Health Policy (New. York).*, vol. 90, no. 2–3, pp. 133–139, May 2009, doi: 10.1016/j.healthpol.2008.09.003

[152] J.-L. Tang, B.-Y. Liu, and K.-W. Ma, "Traditional Chinese medicine," *Lancet*, vol. 372, no. 9654, pp. 1938–1940, Dec. 2008, doi: 10.1016/S0140-6736(08)61354-9

[153] T. Jiang and J. Li, "Review on the systems biology research of Yin-deficiency-heat syndrome in traditional Chinese medicine," *Anat. Rec.*, vol. 306, pp. 2939–2944, Jan. 2020, doi: 10.1002/ar.24354

[154] G. Maciocia, "The practice of Chinese medicine," *Soc. Mar. Q.*, vol. 1, no. 1. p. 1741, 1994, doi: 10.1080/15245004.1994.9960942

[155] K. Bilton, L. Hammer, and C. Zaslawski, "Contemporary Chinese pulse diagnosis: A modern interpretation of an ancient and traditional method," *J. Acupunct. Meridian Stud.*, vol. 6, no. 5, pp. 227–233, Oct. 2013, doi: 10.1016/j.jams.2013.04.002

[156] L. I. Hammer, *Chinese Pulse Diagnosis a Contemporary Chinese Pulse Diagnosis, revised edition, 2005*. Eastland Press.

[157] L. I. Hammer and H. Rotte, *Chinese Herbal Medicine, , 2013*. Georg Thieme Verlag.

[158] M. M. Pandey, S. Rastogi, and A. K. S. Rawat, "Indian traditional ayur-vedic system of medicine and nutritional supplementation," *Evidence-Based Complement. Altern. Med.*, vol. 2013, pp. 1–12, 2013, doi: 10.1155/2013/376327

[159] A. Chopra and V. V Doiphode, "Ayurvedic medicine: Core concept, thera-peutic principles, and current relevance," *Med. Clin. North Am.*, vol. 86, no. 1, pp. 75–89, Jan. 2002, doi: 10.1016/S0025-7125(03)00073-7

[160] P. J. Mills et al., "Relationships among classifications of ayurvedic medicine diagnostics for imbalances and western measures of psychological states: An exploratory study," *J. Ayurveda Integr. Med.*, vol. 10, no. 3, pp. 198–202, Jul. 2019, doi: 10.1016/j.jaim.2018.02.001

[161] B. Prasher et al., "Whole genome expression and biochemical correlates of extreme constitutional types defined in Ayurveda," *J. Transl. Med.*, vol. 6, no. 1, p. 48, 2008, doi: 10.1186/1479-5876-6-48

[162] B. V. Manyam and A. Kumar, "Ayurvedic constitution (Prakruti) identifies risk factor of developing Parkinson's disease," *J. Altern. Complement. Med.*, vol. 19, no. 7, pp. 644–649, Jul. 2013, doi: 10.1089/acm.2011.0809

[163] S. M. S. Samarakoon, B. Ravishankar, and H. Chandola, "Effect of dietary, social, and lifestyle determinants of accelerated aging and its common clinical presentation: A survey study," *AYU (An Int. Q. J. Res. Ayurveda)*, vol. 32, no. 3, p. 315, 2011, doi: 10.4103/0974-8520.93906

[164] P. V. G. Kumar, S. Deshpande, and H. R. Nagendra, "Traditional practices and recent advances in Nadi Pariksha: A comprehensive review," *J. Ayurveda Integr. Med.*, vol. 10, no. 4, pp. 308–315, Oct. 2019, doi: 10.1016/j.jaim.2017.10.007

[165] S. Mahesh, M. Manivannan, and T. Anandan, "Three radial artery pulse sensor design for siddha based disease diagnosis." Inter. J. of Sys., Cybe.r and Info. (IJSCI), pp. 19–23, July 2008. Institute of Scientific and Technical Education (ISTE), India.

[166] V. D. Lad, *Secrets of the Pulse: The Ancient Art of Ayurvedic Pulse Diagnosis.* Motilal Banarsidass, 2005.

[167] C. Y. Chung, Y. F. Chung, Y. W. Chu, and C. H. Luo, "Spatial feature extraction from wrist pulse signals," in *ICOT 2013 1st International Conference Orange Technologies*, pp. 1–4, 2013, doi: 10.1109/ICOT.2013.6521142

[168] D. Rangaprakash and D. Narayana Dutt, "Study of wrist pulse signals using time domain spatial features," *Comput. Electr. Eng.*, vol. 45, pp. 100–107, 2015, doi: 10.1016/j.compeleceng.2014.12.016

[169] D.-Y. Zhang, W.-M. Zuo, D. Zhang, H.-Z. Zhang, and N.-M. Li, "Wrist blood flow signal-based computerized pulse diagnosis using spatial and spectrum features," *J. Biomed. Sci. Eng.*, vol. 3, no. April, pp. 361–366, 2010, doi: 10.4236/jbise.2010.34050

[170] J. P. Curtis et al., "The pre-hospital electrocardiogram and time to reperfusion in patients with acute myocardial infarction, 2000-2002. Findings from the National Registry of Myocardial Infarction-4," *J. Am. Coll. Cardiol.*, vol. 47, no. 8, pp. 1544–1552, 2006, doi: 10.1016/j.jacc.2005.10.077

[171] B. J. Drew and M. Funk, "Practice standards for ECG monitoring in hospital settings: Executive summary and guide for implementation," *Crit. Care Nurs. Clin. North Am.*, vol. 18, no. 2, pp. 157–168, 2006, doi: 10.1016/j.ccell.2006.01.007

[172] L. F. Lyckhage, M. L. Hansen, K. Procida, and T. Wienecke, "Prehospital continuous ECG is valuable for very early detection of atrial fibrillation in patients with acute stroke," *J. Stroke Cerebrovasc. Dis.*, vol. 29, no. 9, 105014, 2020, doi: 10.1016/j.jstrokecerebrovasdis.2020.105014

[173] K. Vandecasteele et al., "Automated epileptic seizure detection based on wearable ECG and PPG in a hospital environment," *Sensors (Switzerland)*, vol. 17, no. 10, pp. 1–12, 2017, doi: 10.3390/s17102338

[174] P. Paolisso et al., "P663 Is echocardiogram alone sufficient for cardiac masses characterization?," *Eur. Hear. J. Cardiovasc. Imag.*, vol. 21, no. Supplement_1, p. 663, 2020, doi: 10.1093/ehjci/jez319.343

[175] W. Toussaint, D. Van Veen, C. Irwin, Y. Nachmany, M. Barreiro-Perez, E. Díaz-Peláez, S. Guerreiro de Sousa, L. Millán, P. L. Sánchez, A. Sánchez-Puente, J. Sampedro-Gómez, P. I. Dorado-Díaz, and V. Vicente-Palacios, "Design considerations for high impact, automated echocardiogram analysis," 2020. Available: http://arxiv.org/abs/2006.06292

[176] R. Hindocha et al., "A minimum dataset for a level 1 echocardiogram: a guideline protocol from the British Society of Echocardiography," *Echo Res. Pract.*, vol. 7, no. 2, pp. G51–G58, 2020, doi: 10.1530/erp-19-0060

[177] N. Gadsbøll et al., "Symptoms and signs of heart failure in patients with myocardial infarction: Reproducibility and relationship to chest X-ray, radionuclide ventriculography and right heart catheterization," *Eur. Heart J.*, vol. 10, no. 11, pp. 1017–1028, Nov. 1989, doi: http://dx.doi.org/10.1093/oxfordjournals.eurheartj.a059414

[178] T. Mota, H. Morais, F. Matias, and C. Costa, "The value of the electrocardiogram and chest X-ray for confirming or refuting a suspected diagnosis of heart failure in the community Candida," *Eur. J. Heart Fail.*, vol. 6, no. 6, pp. 821–822, 2004, doi: 10.1016/j.ejheart.2004.09.002

[179] P. McKavanagh et al., "A comparison of cardiac computerized tomography and exercise stress electrocardiogramtest for the investigation of stable chest pain: The clinical results of the CAPP randomized prospective trial," *Eur. Heart J. Cardiovasc. Imaging,* vol. 16, no. 4, pp. 441–448, 2015, doi: 10.1093/ehjci/jeu284

[180] Y. Dori et al., "X-ray magnetic resonance fusion to internal markers and utility in congenital heart disease catheterization," *Circ. Cardiovasc. Imaging,* vol. 4, no. 4, pp. 415–424, 2011, doi: 10.1161/CIRCIMAGING.111. 963868

[181] S. Oparil and C. E. Lewis, "Should patients with cardiovascular risk factors receive intensive treatment of hypertension to <120/80 mm Hg Target?: A protagonist view from the SPRINT Trial (Systolic Blood Pressure Intervention Trial)," *Circulation*, vol. 134, no. 18, pp. 1308–1310, 2016, doi: 10.1161/CIRCULATIONAHA.116.023263

[182] Y. Ma et al., "Evaluating the accuracy of an aneroid sphygmomanometer in a clinical trial setting," *Am. J. Hypertens.*, vol. 22, no. 3, pp. 263–266, 2009, doi: 10.1038/ajh.2008.338

[183] R. Mastouri, S. G. Sawada, and J. Mahenthiran, "Current noninvasive imaging techniques for detection of coronary artery disease," *Expert Rev. Cardiovasc. Ther.*, vol. 8, no. 1, pp. 77–91, Jan. 2010, doi: 10.1586/erc.09.164

[184] E. Escolar, "New imaging techniques for diagnosing coronary artery disease," *Can. Med. Assoc. J.*, vol. 174, no. 4, pp. 487–495, Feb. 2006, doi: 10.1503/cmaj.050925

[185] M. Tavakol, S. Ashraf, and S. J. Brener, "Risks and complications of coronary angiography: A comprehensive review," *Glob. J. Health Sci.*, vol. 4, no. 1, Dec. 2011, doi: 10.5539/gjhs.v4n1p65

[186] W. J. Verberk, H. Cheng, L.-C. Huang, C.-M. Lin, Y.-P. Teng, and C.-H. Chen, "Practical suitability of a stand-alone oscillometric central blood pressure monitor: A review of the microlife WatchBP office central," *Pulse*, vol. 3, no. 3–4, pp. 205–216, 2016, doi: 10.1159/000443771

[187] J. E. Lewis, P. Williams, and J. H. Davies, "Non-invasive assessment of peripheral arterial disease: Automated ankle brachial index measurement and pulse volume analysis compared to duplex scan," *SAGE open Med.*, vol. 4, 2050312116659088, 2016, doi: 10.1177/2050312116659088

[188] Y. Watanabe et al., "Ankle-brachial index, toe-brachial index, and pulse volume recording in healthy young adults," *Ann. Vasc. Dis.*, vol. 8, no. 3, pp. 227–235, 2015, doi: 10.3400/avd.oa.15-00056

[189] R. E. D. Climie, M. G. Schultz, S. B. Nikolic, K. D. K. Ahuja, J. W. Fell, and J. E. Sharman, "Validity and reliability of central blood pressure estimated by upper arm oscillometric cuff pressure.," *Am. J. Hypertens.*, vol. 25, no. 4, pp. 414–420, Apr. 2012, doi: 10.1038/ajh.2011.238.

[190] C. U. Choi et al., "Differing effects of aging on central and peripheral blood pressures and pulse wave velocity: a direct intraarterial study.," *J. Hypertens.*, vol. 28, no. 6, pp. 1252–1260, Jun. 2010, doi: 10.1097/HJH.0b013e328337dad6

[191] E. J. Kroeker and E. H. Wood, "Comparison of simultaneously recorded central and peripheral arterial pressure pulses during rest, exercise and tilted position in man," *Circ. Res.*, vol. 3, no. 6, pp. 623–632, 1955, doi: 10.1161/01.RES.3.6.623

[192] A. L. Pauca, S. L. Wallenhaupt, N. D. Kon, and W. Y. Tucker, "Does radial artery pressure accurately reflect aortic pressure?," *Chest*, vol. 102, no. 4, pp. 1193–1198, Oct. 1992, doi: 10.1378/chest.102.4.1193

[193] A. P. Avolio et al., "Role of pulse pressure amplification in arterial hypertension: Experts' opinion and review of the data" *Hypertens. (Dallas, Tex. 1979)*, vol. 54, no. 2, pp. 375–383, Aug. 2009, doi: 10.1161/HYPERTENSIONAHA.109.134379

[194] C. Vlachopoulos, K. Aznaouridis, M. F. O'Rourke, M. E. Safar, K. Baou, and C. Stefanadis, "Prediction of cardiovascular events and all-cause mortality with central haemodynamics: A systematic review and meta-analysis," *Eur. Heart J.*, vol. 31, no. 15, pp. 1865–1871, Aug. 2010, doi: 10.1093/eurheartj/ehq024

[195] S. Theilade, T. W. Hansen, and P. Rossing, "Central hemodynamics are associated with cardiovascular disease and albuminuria in type 1 diabetes," *Am. J. Hypertens.*, vol. 27, no. 9, pp. 1152–1159, 2014, doi: 10.1093/ajh/hpu030

[196] R. Pini et al., "Central but not brachial blood pressure predicts cardiovascular events in an unselected geriatric population. The ICARe Dicomano study," *J. Am. Coll. Cardiol.*, vol. 51, no. 25, pp. 2432–2439, 2008, doi: 10.1016/j.jacc.2008.03.031

[197] K. Wang, H. Cheng, S. Chuang, and H. A. Spurgeon, "Central or peripheral systolic or pulse pressure: Which best relates to target-organs and future," *J Hypertens*, vol. 27, no. 201, pp. 461–467, 2011.

[198] M. J. Roman et al., "Central pressure more strongly relates to vascular disease and outcome than does brachial pressure: the Strong Heart Study," *Hypertens. (Dallas, Tex. 1979)*, vol. 50, no. 1, pp. 197–203, Jul. 2007, doi: 10.1161/ HYPERTENSIONAHA.107.089078

[199] P. Jankowski et al., "Pulsatile but not steady component of blood pressure predicts cardiovascular events in coronary patients," *Hypertension*, vol. 51, no. 4, pp. 848–855, Apr. 2008, doi: 10.1161/HYPERTENSIONAHA.107.101725

[200] A. Benetos et al., "Mortality and cardiovascular events are best predicted by low central/peripheral pulse pressure amplification but not by high blood pressure levels in elderly nursing home subjects: The PARTAGE (Predictive Values of Blood Pressure and Arterial Stiffness Institutionalized Very Aged Population) study," *J. Am. Coll. Cardiol.*, vol. 60, no. 16, pp. 1503–1511, 2012, doi: 10.1016/j.jacc.2012.04.055

[201] M. E. Safar et al., "Central pulse pressure and mortality in end-stage renal disease," *Hypertension (Dallas, Tex. 1979)*, vol. 39, no. 3, pp. 735–738, Mar. 2002, doi: 10.1161/hy0202.098325

[202] A. Kollias, S. Lagou, M. E. Zeniodi, N. Boubouchairopoulou, and G. S. Stergiou, "Association of central versus brachial blood pressure with target-organ damage: Systematic review and meta-analysis," *Hypertension*, vol. 67, no. 1, pp. 183–190, 2016, doi: 10.1161/HYPERTENSIONAHA.115.06066

[203] B. Williams et al., "Differential impact of blood pressure-lowering drugs on central aortic pressure and clinical outcomes: Principal results of the Conduit Artery Function Evaluation (CAFE) study," *Circulation*, vol. 113, no. 9, pp. 1213–1225, 2006, doi: 10.1161/CIRCULATIONAHA.105.595496

[204] T. Papaioannou, A. Protogerou, K. Stamatelopoulos, M. Vavuranakis, and C. Stefanadis, "Non-invasive methods and techniques for central blood pressure estimation: Procedures, validation, reproducibility and limitations," *Curr. Pharm. Des.*, vol. 15, no. 3, pp. 245–253, 2009, doi: 10.2174/ 138161209787354203

[205] M. Karamanoglu, M. F. O'Rourke, A. P. Avolio, and R. P. Kelly, "An analysis of the relationship between central aortic and peripheral upper limb pressure waves in man," *Eur. Heart J.*, vol. 14, no. 2, pp. 160–167, Feb. 1993, doi: 10.1093/eurheartj/14.2.160

[206] B. Fetics, E. Nevo, C.-H. Chen, and D. A. Kass, "Parametric model derivation of transfer function for noninvasive estimation of aortic pressure by radial tonometry," *IEEE Trans. Biomed. Eng.*, vol. 46, no. 6, pp. 698–706, Jun. 1999, doi: 10.1109/10.764946

[207] S. A. Hope, I. T. Meredith, D. Tay, and J. D. Cameron, "Generalizability??? of a radial-aortic transfer function for the derivation of central aortic waveform parameters," *J. Hypertens.*, vol. 25, no. 9, pp. 1812–1820, Sep. 2007, doi: 10.1097/HJH.0b013e328277595d

[208] S. A. Hope, I. T. Meredith, and J. D. Cameron, "Arterial transfer functions and the reconstruction of central aortic waveforms: Myths, controversies

and misconceptions," *J. Hypertens.*, vol. 26, no. 1, pp. 4–7, Jan. 2008, doi: 10.1097/HJH.0b013e3282f0c9f5

[209] M. F. O'Rourke, "Mechanical principles. Arterial stiffness and wave reflection," *Pathol. Biol. (Paris).*, vol. 47, no. 6, pp. 623–633, Jun. 1999. Available: http://europepmc.org/abstract/MED/10472073

[210] K. C. Peebles, I. Tan, M. T. D. Cook, D. A. Theobald, A. P. Avolio, and M. Butlin, "Interarm differences in brachial blood pressure and their effect on the derivation on central aortic blood pressure," *Artery Res.*, vol. 26, no. 2, pp. 89–96, 2020, doi: 10.2991/artres.k.200201.002

[211] A. T. Butt, Y. A. Abakr, and K. B. Mustapha, "Blood flow modeling to improve cardiovascular diagnostics: Application of a GTF to predict central aortic pressure using a 1-D model," *Int. J. Eng. Technol.*, vol. 7, no. 4.26, p. 146, Nov. 2018, doi: 10.14419/ijet.v7i4.26.22156

[212] T. G. Papaioannou et al., "Transmission of calibration errors (input) by generalized transfer functions to the aortic pressures (output) at different hemodynamic states," *Int. J. Cardiol.*, vol. 110, no. 1, pp. 46–52, Jun. 2006, doi: 10.1016/j.ijcard.2005.07.014

[213] S. So¨derstro¨m, G. Nyberg, M. F. O'Rourke, J. Sellgren, and J. Pontén, "Can a clinically useful aortic pressure wave be derived from a radial pressure wave?," *Br. J. Anaesth.*, vol. 88, no. 4, pp. 481–488, Apr. 2002, doi: 10.1093/bja/88.4.481

[214] D. Gallagher, A. Adji, and M. F. O'Rourke, "Validation of the transfer function technique for generating central from peripheral upper limb pressure waveform," *Am. J. Hypertens.*, vol. 17, no. 11, pp. 1059–1067, 2004, doi: 10.1016/j.amjhyper.2004.05.027

[215] G. C. Cloud, C. Rajkumar, J. Kooner, J. Cooke, and C. J. Bulpitt, "Estimation of central aortic pressure by SphygmoCor requires intra-arterial peripheral pressures," *Clin. Sci. (Lond).*, vol. 105, no. 2, pp. 219–225, Aug. 2003, doi: 10.1042/CS20030012

[216] T. E. Strandberg and K. Pitkala, "What is the most important component of blood pressure: Systolic, diastolic or pulse pressure?," *Curr. Opin. Nephrol. Hypertens.*, vol. 12, no. 3, pp. 293–297, May 2003, doi: 10.1097/00041552-200305000-00011

[217] M. Gao, W. C. Rose, B. Fetics, D. A. Kass, C. H. Chen, and R. Mukkamala, "A simple adaptive transfer function for deriving the central blood pressure waveform from a radial blood pressure waveform," *Sci. Rep.*, vol. 6, no. August, pp. 1–9, 2016, doi: 10.1038/srep33230

[218] Y. Yao et al., "Validation of an adaptive transfer function method to estimate the aortic pressure waveform," *IEEE J. Biomed. Heal. Informatics*, vol. 21, no. 6, pp. 1599–1606, 2017, doi: 10.1109/JBHI.2016.2636223

[219] G. Swamy, D. Xu, N. B. Olivier, and R. Mukkamala, "An adaptive transfer function for deriving the aortic pressure waveform from a peripheral artery pressure waveform," *Am. J. Physiol. Hear. Circ. Physiol.*, vol. 297, no. 5, pp. 1956–1963, 2009, doi: 10.1152/ajpheart.00155.2009

[220] A. L. Pauca, N. D. Kon, and M. F. O'Rourke, "The second peak of the radial artery pressure wave represents aortic systolic pressure in hypertensive and

elderly patients," *Br. J. Anaesth.*, vol. 92, no. 5, pp. 651–657, May 2004, doi: 10.1093/bja/aeh121

[221] A. Guilcher, S. Brett, S. Munir, B. Clapp, and P. J. Chowienczyk, "Estimating central SBP from the peripheral pulse: Influence of waveform analysis and calibration error," *J. Hypertens.*, vol. 29, no. 7, pp. 1357–1366, Jul. 2011, doi: 10.1097/HJH.0b013e3283479070

[222] W. B. Kannel, D. McGee, and T. Gordon, "A general cardiovascular risk profile: The Framingham study," *Am. J. Cardiol.*, vol. 38, no. 1, pp. 46–51, Jul. 1976, doi: 10.1016/0002-9149(76)90061-8

[223] A. Menotti, P. E. Puddu, and M. Lanti, "Comparison of the Framingham risk function-based coronary chart with risk function from an Italian population study," *Eur. Heart J.*, vol. 21, no. 5, pp. 365–370, 2000, doi: 10.1053/euhj.1999.1864

[224] R. M. Conroy et al., "Estimation of ten-year risk of fatal cardiovascular disease in Europe: The SCORE project," *Eur. Heart J.*, vol. 24, no. 11, pp. 987–1003, 2003, doi: 10.1016/S0195-668X(03)00114-3

[225] D. B. Panagiotakos, A. P. Fitzgerald, C. Pitsavos, A. Pipilis, I. Graham, and C. Stefanadis, "Statistical modelling of 10-year fatal cardiovascular disease risk in Greece: The HellenicSCORE (a calibration of the ESC SCORE project)," *Hell. J. Cardiol.*, vol. 48, no. 2, pp. 55–63, 2007.

[226] A. C. Dimopoulos et al., "Machine learning methodologies versus cardiovascular risk scores, in predicting disease risk," *BMC Med. Res. Methodol.*, vol. 18, no. 1, pp. 1–11, 2018, doi: 10.1186/s12874-018-0644-1

[227] D. Panagiotakos, "Health measurement scales: Methodological issues," *Open Cardiovasc. Med. J.*, vol. 3, no. 1, pp. 160–165, 2009, doi: 10.2174/1874192400903010160

[228] M. T. Cooney, H. C. Cooney, A. Dudina, and I. M. Graham, "Total cardiovascular disease risk assessment," *Curr. Opin. Cardiol.*, vol. 26, no. 5, pp. 429–437, Sep. 2011, doi: 10.1097/HCO.0b013e3283499f06

[229] I. M. Graham, M.-T. Cooney, A. Dudina, and S. Squarta, "What is my risk of developing cardiovascular disease?," *Eur. J. Cardiovasc. Prev. Rehabil.*, vol. 16, no. 2_suppl, pp. S2–S7, Aug. 2009, doi: 10.1097/01.hjr.0000359226.50399.59

[230] R. B. D'Agostino, S. Grundy, L. M. Sullivan, and P. Wilson, "Validation of the Framingham coronary heart disease prediction scores," *Jama*, vol. 286, no. 2, p. 180, 2001, doi: 10.1001/jama.286.2.180

[231] B. Y. Enyew and Z. G. Asfaw, "Comparison of survival models and assessment of risk factors for survival of cardiovascular patients at Addis Ababa Cardiac Center, Ethiopia: A retrospective study," *Afr. Health Sci.*, vol. 21, no. 3, pp. 1201–1213, 2021, doi: 10.4314/ahs.v21i3.29

[232] C. El-Hajj and P. A. Kyriacou, "A review of machine learning techniques in photoplethysmography for the non-invasive cuff-less measurement of blood pressure," *Biomed. Signal Process. Control*, vol. 58, p. 101870, 2020, doi: 10.1016/j.bspc.2020.101870

[233] I. Kononenko, "Machine learning for medical diagnosis: History, state of the art and perspective," *Artif. Intell. Med.*, vol. 23, no. 1, pp. 89–109, 2001, doi: 10.1016/S0933-3657(01)00077-X

[234] I. Yoo et al., "Data mining in healthcare and biomedicine: A survey of the literature," *J. Med. Syst.*, vol. 36, no. 4, pp. 2431–2448, 2012, doi: 10.1007/s10916-011-9710-5

[235] K. Kourou, T. P. Exarchos, K. P. Exarchos, M. V. Karamouzis, and D. I. Fotiadis, "Machine learning applications in cancer prognosis and prediction," *Comput. Struct. Biotechnol. J.*, vol. 13, pp. 8–17, 2015, doi: 10.1016/j.csbj.2014.11.005

[236] S. Wang and R. M. Summers, "Machine learning and radiology," *Med. Image Anal.*, vol. 16, no. 5, pp. 933–951, 2012, doi: 10.1016/j.media.2012.02.005

[237] F. Fabris, J. P. de Magalhães, and A. A. Freitas, "A review of supervised machine learning applied to ageing research," *Biogerontology*, vol. 18, no. 2, pp. 171–188, 2017, doi: 10.1007/s10522-017-9683-y

[238] S. F. Weng, J. Reps, J. Kai, J. M. Garibaldi, and N. Qureshi, "Can Machine-learning improve cardiovascular risk prediction using routine clinical data?," *PLoS One*, vol. 12, no. 4, pp. 1–14, 2017, doi: 10.1371/journal.pone.0174944

[239] H. Liu, "Book review: Machine Learning, Neural and Statistical Classification Edited by D. Michie, D.J. Spiegelhalter and C.C. Taylor (Ellis Horwood Limited, 1994)," *ACM SIGART Bull.*, vol. 7, no. 1, pp. 16–17, Jan. 1996, doi: 10.1145/230062.1066049

[240] M. Minsky, Theory of neural-analog reinforcement systems and their application to brain model problems (Ph.D. dissertation, Princeton University), 1954.

[241] C. M. Shufflebarger, "What is neutral network?," *Ann. Emerg. Med.*, vol. 21, no. 12, pp. 1461–1462, Dec. 1992, doi: 10.1016/S0196-0644(05)80060-5

[242] D. E. Rumelhart, G. E. Hinton, and R. J. Williams, "Learning internal representations by error propagation," in *Parallel Distributed Processing: Explorations in the Microstructure of Cognition, Vol. 1: Foundations*, 1986, pp. 318–362. MIT Press.

[243] D. E. Rumelhart, G. E. Hinton, and R. J. Williams, "Learning representations by back-propagating errors," *Nature*, vol. 323, no. 6088, pp. 533–536, Oct. 1986, doi: 10.1038/323533a0

[244] D. Itchhaporia, P. B. Snow, R. J. Almassy, and W. J. Oetgen, "Artificial neural networks: Current status in cardiovascular medicine," *J. Am. Coll. Cardiol.*, vol. 28, no. 2, pp. 515–521, 1996, doi: 10.1016/S0735-1097(96)00174-X

[245] J. A. Scott and E. L. Palmer, "Neural network analysis of ventilation-perfusion lung scans.," *Radiology*, vol. 186, no. 3, pp. 661–664, Mar. 1993, doi: 10.1148/radiology.186.3.8430170

[246] H. Ebell, "Artificial neural networks for predicting failure to survive following in-hospital cardiopulmonary resuscitation," *J. Fam. Pract.* vol. 3, no. 3, pp. 297–303, 1993.

[247] R. Poli, S. Cagnoni, R. Livi, G. Coppini, and G. Valli, "A neural network expert system for diagnosing and treating hypertension," *Computer (Long. Beach. Calif).*, vol. 24, no. 3, pp. 64–71, Mar. 1991, doi: 10.1109/2.73514

[248] M. Akay, "Noninvasive diagnosis of coronary artery disease using a neural network algorithm," *Biol. Cybern.*, vol. 67, no. 4, pp. 361–367, Aug. 1992, doi: 10.1007/BF02414891

[249] P. W. Macfarlane, B. Devine, S. Latif, S. McLaughlin, D. B. Shoat, and M. P. Watts, "Methodology of ECG interpretation in the Glasgow program.," *Methods Inf. Med.*, vol. 29, no. 4, pp. 354–361, Sep. 1990.

[250] P. W. Macfarlane, "A brief history of computer-assisted electrocardiography," *Methods Inf. Med.*, vol. 29, no. 04, pp. 272–281, Feb. 1990, doi: 10.1055/s-0038-1634791

[251] G. Bortolan, R. Degani, and J. L. Willems, "Design of neural networks for classification of electrocardiographic signals," in *Proceedings of the Twelfth Annual International Conference of the IEEE Engineering in Medicine and Biology Society*, pp. 1467–1468, 1990, doi: 10.1109/IEMBS.1990.691842

[252] L. Edenbrandt, B. Devine, and P. W. Macfarlane, "Classification of electrocardiographic ST-T segments – human expert vs artificial neural network," *Eur. Heart J.*, vol. 14, no. 4, pp. 464–468, Apr. 1993, doi: 10.1093/eurheartj/14.4.464

[253] B. Hedén, L. Edenbrandt, W. K. Haisty, and O. Pahlm, "Artificial neural networks for the electrocardiographic diagnosis of healed myocardial infarction," *Am. J. Cardiol.*, vol. 74, no. 1, pp. 5–8, Jul. 1994, doi: 10.1016/0002-9149(94)90482-0

[254] W. R. M. Dassen et al., "An artificial neural network to localize atrioventricular accessory pathways in patients suffering from the Wolff-Parkinson-White Syndrome," *Pacing Clin. Electrophysiol.*, vol. 13, no. 12, pp. 1792–1796, Dec. 1990, doi: 10.1111/j.1540-8159.1990.tb06892.x

[255] K. Kario et al., "Development of a new ICT-based multisensor blood pressure monitoring system for use in hemodynamic biomarker-initiated anticipation medicine for cardiovascular disease: The National Impact Program Project," *Prog. Cardiovasc. Dis.*, vol. 60, no. 3, pp. 435–449, 2017, doi: 10.1016/j.pcad.2017.10.002

[256] Z. Shen, R. W. Jones, and T. Alberti, "Detecting the risk factors of coronary heart disease by use of neural networks," in *Proceedings of Annual Conference of the IEEE Engineering in Medicine Biology*, vol. 15, no. pt 1, pp. 277–278, 1993, doi: 10.1109/iembs.1993.978541

[257] S. U. Amin, K. Agarwal, and R. Beg, "Genetic neural network based data mining in prediction of heart disease using risk factors," in *2013 IEEE Conference on Information and Communication Technology* 2013, no. February, pp. 1227–1231, 2013, doi: 10.1109/CICT.2013.6558288

[258] J. S. Sonawane and D. R. Patil, "Prediction of heart disease using learning vector quantization algorithm," in *Proceedings of 2014 Conference on IT Business, Industry and Government by CSI Big Data* 2014, pp. 0–4, 2014, doi: 10.1109/CSIBIG.2014.7056973

[259] S. Bashir, U. Qamar, and M. Y. Javed, "An ensemble based decision support framework for intelligent heart disease diagnosis," in *International Conference on Information Society and Technology*, 2014, no. January, pp. 259–264, 2015, doi: 10.1109/i-Society.2014.7009056

[260] M. G. Feshki and O. S. Shijani, "Improving the heart disease diagnosis by evolutionary algorithm of PSO and feed forward neural network," in *2016 Artificial Intelligence and Robotics IRANOPEN* 2016, pp. 48–53, 2016, doi: 10.1109/RIOS.2016.7529489

[261] S. Carbone, J. M. Canada, H. E. Billingsley, M. S. Siddiqui, A. Elagizi, and C. J. Lavie, "Obesity paradox in cardiovascular disease: Where do we stand?," *Vasc. Health Risk Manag.*, vol. 15, pp. 89–100, 2019, doi: 10.2147/VHRM.S168946

[262] S. Carbone, C. J. Lavie, and R. Arena, "Obesity and heart failure: Focus on the obesity paradox," *Mayo Clin. Proc.*, vol. 92, no. 2, pp. 266–279, 2017, doi: 10.1016/j.mayocp.2016.11.001

[263] A. Elagizi et al., "An overview and update on obesity and the obesity paradox in cardiovascular diseases," *Prog. Cardiovasc. Dis.*, vol. 61, no. 2, pp. 142–150, 2018, doi: 10.1016/j.pcad.2018.07.003

[264] C. J. Lavie et al., "Obesity and prevalence of cardiovascular diseases and prognosis-The obesity paradox updated," *Prog. Cardiovasc. Dis.*, vol. 58, no. 5, pp. 537–547, 2016, doi: 10.1016/j.pcad.2016.01.008

[265] R. Stamler, C. E. Ford, and J. Stamler, "Why do lean hypertensives have higher mortality rates than other hypertensives? Findings of the hypertension detection and follow-up program," *Hypertension*, vol. 17, no. 4, pp. 553–564, 1991, doi: 10.1161/01.HYP.17.4.553

[266] A. Jayedi and S. Shab-Bidar, "Nonlinear dose–response association between body mass index and risk of all-cause and cardiovascular mortality in patients with hypertension: A meta-analysis," *Obes. Res. Clin. Pract.*, vol. 12, no. 1, pp. 16–28, 2018, doi: 10.1016/j.orcp.2018.01.002

[267] A. O. Badheka et al., "Influence of obesity on outcomes in atrial fibrillation: Yet another obesity paradox," *Am. J. Med.*, vol. 123, no. 7, pp. 646–651, Jul. 2010, doi: 10.1016/j.amjmed.2009.11.026

[268] R. K. Sandhu et al., "The 'obesity paradox' in atrial fibrillation: Observations from the ARISTOTLE (Apixaban for Reduction in Stroke and Other Thromboembolic Events in Atrial Fibrillation) trial," *Eur. Heart J.*, vol. 37, no. 38, pp. 2869–2878, 2016, doi: 10.1093/eurheartj/ehw124

[269] M. Agarwal, S. Agrawal, L. Garg, and C. J. Lavie, "Relation between obesity and survival in patients hospitalized for pulmonary arterial hypertension (from a Nationwide Inpatient Sample Database 2003 to 2011)," *Am. J. Cardiol.*, vol. 120, no. 3, pp. 489–493, Aug. 2017, doi: 10.1016/j.amjcard.2017.04.051

[270] M. Brida et al., "Body mass index in adult congenital heart disease," *Heart*, vol. 103, no. 16, pp. 1250–1257, Aug. 2017, doi: 10.1136/heartjnl-2016-310571

[271] M. H. Olsen et al., "A call to action and a lifecourse strategy to address the global burden of raised blood pressure on current and future generations: The Lancet Commission on hypertension," *Lancet*, vol. 388, no. 10060, pp. 2665–2712, Nov. 2016, doi: 10.1016/S0140-6736(16)31134-5

[272] M. F. O'Rourke, "Hypertension is a myth; high(er) arterial pressure is the problem.," *Aust. N. Z. J. Med.*, vol. 14, no. 1, pp. 69–70, Feb. 1984, doi: 10.1111/j.1445-5994.1984.tb03594.x

[273] A. E. Doyle, "Hypertension: The realities.," *Aust. N. Z. J. Med.*, vol. 13, no. 2, pp. 185–186, Apr. 1983, doi: 10.1111/j.1445-5994.1983.tb02684.x

[274] A. Avolio, "Central aortic blood pressure and cardiovascular risk: A paradigm shift?," *Hypertension*, vol. 51, no. 6, pp. 1470–1471, 2008, doi: 10.1161/ HYPERTENSIONAHA.107.108910

[275] W. W. Nichols, M. F. O'Rourke, and D. A. McDonald, *McDonald's Blood Flow in Arteries: Theoretical, Experimental, And Clinical Principles,* 2005. Hodder Arnold.

[276] N. Westerhof, P. Sipkema, G. C. V. D. Bos, and G. Elzinga, "Forward and backward waves in the arterial system," *Cardiovasc. Res.*, vol. 6, no. 6, pp. 648–656, Nov. 1972, doi: 10.1093/cvr/6.6.648

[277] J. C. Kovacic, N. Mercader, M. Torres, M. Boehm, and V. Fuster, "Epithelial-to-mesenchymal and endothelial-to-mesenchymal transition," Circulation, vol. 125, no. 14, pp. 1795–1808, Apr. 2012, doi: 10.1161/ CIRCULATIONAHA.111.040352

[278] H. Eom et al., "End-to-end deep learning architecture for continuous blood pressure estimation using attention mechanism," *Sensors (Switzerland)*, vol. 20, no. 8, pp. 1–20, 2020, doi: 10.3390/s20082338

[279] Q. Chen et al., "A survey on an emerging area: Deep learning for smart city data," *IEEE Trans. Emerg. Top. Comput. Intell.*, vol. 3, no. 5, pp. 392–410, 2019, doi: 10.1109/TETCI.2019.2907718

[280] Y. Lecun, Y. Bengio, and G. Hinton, "Deep learning," *Nature*, vol. 521, no. 7553, pp. 436–444, 2015, doi: 10.1038/nature14539

[281] A. Graves, A. Mohamed, and G. Hinton, "Speech recognition with deep recurrent neural networks,"in *2013 IEEE International Conference on Acoustics, Speech and Signal Processing (ICASSP)*, 2013, pp. 6645–6649, doi: 10.1109/ ICASSP.2013.6638947

[282] K. Greff, R. K. Srivastava, J. Koutnik, B. R. Steunebrink, and J. Schmidhuber, "LSTM: A search space odyssey," in *IEEE Transactions on Neural Networks and Learning Systems*, vol. 28, no. 10, pp. 2222–2232, 2017, doi: 10.1109/ TNNLS.2016.2582924

[283] G. Li, K. Watanabe, H. Anzai, X. Song, A. Qiao, and M. Ohta, "Pulse-wave-pattern classification with a convolutional neural network," *Sci. Rep.*, vol. 9, no. 1, pp. 1–11, 2019, doi: 10.1038/s41598-019-51334-2

[284] G. B. Huang, H. Lee, and E. Learned-Miller, "Learning hierarchical representations for face verification with convolutional deep belief networks," in *Proceedings of the IEEE Computer Society Conference on Computer Vision and Pattern Recognition*, pp. 2518–2525, 2012, doi: 10.1109/ CVPR.2012.6247968

[285] A. Krizhevsky, I. Sutskever, and G. E. Hinton, "ImageNet classification with deep convolutional neural networks," in *Proceedings of the 25th International Conference on Neural Information Processing Systems*, vol. 1, pp. 1097–1105, 2012.

[286] K. Simonyan and A. Zisserman, "Very deep convolutional networks for large-scale image recognition," in *3rd International Conference on Learning Representations, ICLR 2015*, pp. 1–14, 2015.

[287] J. Zhang, P. Liu, F. Zhang, and Q. Song, "CloudNet: Ground-based cloud classification with deep convolutional neural network," *Geophys. Res. Lett.*, vol. 45, no. 16, pp. 8665–8672, 2018, doi: 10.1029/2018GL077787

[288] M. Zubair and J. Kim, *"An automated ECG beat classification system using convolutional neural networks,"* in *2016 6th International Conference on IT Convergence and Security (ICITCS*, 2016, pp. 1–5. Prague, Czech Republic, doi: 10.1109/ICITCS.2016.7740310

[289] D. Li, J. Zhang, Q. Zhang, and X. Wei, "Classification of ECG signals based on 1D convolution neural network," in *2017 IEEE 19th International Conference on e-Health Networking, Applications and Services (Healthcom)*, 2017, pp. 2–7. Dalian, China, doi: 10.1109/HealthCom.2017.8210784

[290] A. Isin and S. Ozdalili, "Cardiac arrhythmia detection using deep learning," *Procedia Comput. Sci.*, vol. 120, pp. 268–275, 2018, doi: 10.1016/j.procs.2017.11.238

[291] P. Rajpurkar, A. Y. Hannun, M. Haghpanahi, C. Bourn, and A. Y. Ng, "Cardiologist-level arrhythmia detection with convolutional neural networks," *arXiv*, 2017, doi: 10.48550/arXiv.1707.01836

[292] U. R. Acharya, H. Fujita, O. S. Lih, Y. Hagiwara, J. H. Tan, and M. Adam, "Automated detection of arrhythmias using different intervals of tachycardia ECG segments with convolutional neural network," *Inf. Sci.*, vol. 405, no. C, pp. 81–90, Sep. 2017, doi: 10.1016/j.ins.2017.04.012

[293] U. R. Acharya, H. Fujita, S. Lih, Y. Hagiwara, J. Hong, and M. Adam, "Application of deep convolutional neural network for automated detection of myocardial infarction using ECG signals," *Inf. Sci. (Ny).*, vol. 415–416, pp. 190–198, 2017, doi: 10.1016/j.ins.2017.06.027

[294] U. R. Acharya, H. Fujita, O. Shu, M. Adam, J. Hong, and C. Kuang, "Knowle dge-Base d Systems Automated detection of coronary artery disease using different durations of ECG segments with convolutional neural network," *Knowledge-Based Syst.*, vol. 132, pp. 62–71, 2017, doi: 10.1016/j.knosys.2017.06.003

[295] Z. Yao, Z. Zhu, and Y. Chen, "Atrial fibrillation detection by multi-scale convolutional neural networks," in *20th International Conference on Information Fusion (Fusion 2017)*, 2017. Xi'an, China, doi: 10.23919/ICIF.2017.8009782

[296] L. Jin and J. Dong, "Classification of normal and abnormal ECG records using lead convolutional neural network and rule inference," vol. 60, no. July, pp. 6–8, 2017, doi: 10.1007/s11432-016-9047-6

[297] M. Wu, E. J. Chang, and T. Chu, "Personalizing a generic ECG heartbeat classification for arrhythmia detection: A deep learning approach," 2018, doi: 10.1109/MIPR.2018.00024

[298] Y. Xia, N. Wulan, K. Wang, and H. Zhang, "Detecting atrial fi brillation by deep convolutional neural networks," *Comput. Biol. Med.*, vol. 93, no. July 2017, pp. 84–92, 2018, doi: 10.1016/j.compbiomed.2017.12.007

[299] U. R. Acharya, H. Fujita, S. L. Oh, Y. Hagiwara, J. H. Tan, M. Adam, and R. S. Tan, "Deep convolutional neural network for the automated diagnosis of congestive heart failure using ECG signals," *Appl. Intell.*, vol. 49, no. 1, pp. 16–27, 2019, doi: 10.1007/s10489-018-1179-1

[300] R. Xiao et al., "Monitoring signi fi cant ST changes through deep learning," *J. Electrocardiol.*, vol. 51, no. 6, pp. S78–S82, 2018, doi: 10.1016/j.jelectrocard.2018.07.026

[301] W. Zhong, L. Liao, X. Guo, and G. Wang, "A deep learning approach for fetal QRS complex detection.," *Physiol. Meas.*, vol. 39, no. 4, 45004, Apr. 2018, doi: 10.1088/1361-6579/aab297

[302] Q. Yao, R. Wang, X. Fan, J. Liu, and Y. Li, "Multi-class arrhythmia detection from 12-lead varied-length ECG using attention-based time-incremental convolutional neural network," vol. 53, no. June 2019, pp. 174–182, 2020, doi: 10.1016/j.inffus.2019.06.024

[303] R. Avanzato and F. Beritelli, "Automatic ECG diagnosis using convolutional neural network," *Electronics*, vol. 9, no. 6, 951, 2020, doi: www.mdpi.com/2079-9292/9/6/951

[304] T. Wang, C. Lu, Y. Sun, M. Yang, C. Liu, and C. Ou, "Automatic ECG classification using continuous wavelet transform and convolutional neural network," *Entropy*, vol. 23, no. 1, 119, pp. 1–13, 2021, doi: 10.3390/e23010119

[305] C. Potes, S. Parvaneh, A. Rahman, and B. Conroy, "Ensemble of feature-based and deep learning-based classifiers for detection of abnormal heart sounds," *Comput. Cardiol.* (2010)., vol. 43, pp. 621–624, 2016, doi: 10.22489/cinc.2016.182-399

[306] H. Ryu, J. Park, and H. Shin, "Classification of heart sound recordings using convolution neural network," *Comput. Cardiol.* (2010)., vol. 43, pp. 1153–1156, 2016, doi: 10.22489/cinc.2016.329-134

[307] J. Rubin, R. Abreu, A. Ganguli, S. Nelaturi, I. Matei, and K. Sricharan, "Classifying heart sound recordings using deep convolutional neural networks and mel-frequency cepstral coefficients," *Comput. Cardiol.* (2010)., vol. 43, pp. 813–816, 2016, doi: 10.22489/cinc.2016.236-175

[308] D. Kucharski, D. Grochala, M. Kajor, and E. Kańtoch, "A deep learning approach for valve defect recognition in heart acoustic signal," in *38th International Conference on Information Systems Architecture and Technology (ISAT 2017)*, pp. 3–14, 2018. Szklarska Poręba, Poland, doi: 10.1007/978-3-319-98813-4_1

[309] J. P. Dominguez-Morales, A. F. Jimenez-Fernandez, M. J. Dominguez-Morales, and G. Jimenez-Moreno, "Deep neural networks for the recognition and classification of heart murmurs using neuromorphic auditory sensors," *IEEE Trans. Biomed. Circuits Syst.*, vol. 12, no. 1, pp. 24–34, 2018, doi: 10.1109/TBCAS.2017.2751545

[310] X. Hu, X. Zhu, J. Xu, D. Xu, and J. Dong, "Wrist pulse signals analysis based on deep convolutional neural networks," in *2014 IEEE Conference on Computational Intelligence in Bioinformatics and Computational Biology (CIBCB)*, 2014, doi: 10.1109/CIBCB.2014.6845525

[311] Y.-J. Moon et al., "Deep learning-based stroke volume estimation outperforms conventional arterial contour method in patients with hemodynamic instability," *J. Clin. Med.*, vol. 8, no. 9, 1419, 2019, doi: 10.3390/jcm8091419

[312] S. Shimazaki, H. Kawanaka, H. Ishikawa, K. Inoue, and K. Oguri, "Cuffless blood pressure estimation from only the waveform of photoplethysmography

using CNN," in *Proceedings of the 25th Annual International Conference on the IEEE Engineering Medicine and Biology Society*, pp. 5042–5045, 2019. Berlin, Germany. doi: 10.1109/EMBC.2019.8856706

[313] E. M. M. Besterman, "William Harvey and his discovery of the circulation of the blood," *West Indian Med. J.*, vol. 53, no. 6, pp. 425–426, 2004, doi: 10.1002/clc.4960080411

[314] J. T. Ottesen, "Valveless pumping in a fluid-filled closed elastic tube-system: one-dimensional theory with experimental validation," *J. Math. Biol.*, vol. 46, no. 4, pp. 309–332, Apr. 2003, doi: 10.1007/s00285-002-0179-1

[315] A. Quarteroni and L. Formaggia, *"Mathematical modelling and numerical simulation of the cardiovascular system,"* MOX, Mathematics Department Politecnico di Milano, Italy and Institute of Mathematics EPFL, Lausanne, Switzerland, 2002.

[316] M. A. Fernández, "Coupling schemes for incompressible fluid-structure interaction: implicit, semi-implicit and explicit," *SeMA J.*, vol. 55, no. 1, pp. 59–108, Sep. 2011, doi: 10.1007/BF03322593

[317] L. Formaggia and A. Veneziani, "Reduced and multiscale models for the human cardiovascular system," *Lect. Notes VKI Lect. Ser.*, no. May, p. 120, 2003, doi: 10.13140/RG.2.1.3668.8088

[318] J. R. Cebral, M. A. Castro, J. E. Burgess, R. S. Pergolizzi, M. J. Sheridan, and C. M. Putman, "Characterization of cerebral aneurysms for assessing risk of rupture by using patient-specific computational hemodynam ics models," *Am. J. Neuroradiol.*, vol. 26, no. 10, pp. 2550 LP–2559, Nov. 2005. Available: www.ajnr.org/content/26/10/2550.abstract

[319] C. A. Taylor and D. A. Steinman, "Image-based modeling of blood flow and vessel wall dynamics: Applications, methods and future directions," *Ann. Biomed. Eng.*, vol. 38, no. 3, pp. 1188–1203, Mar. 2010, doi: 10.1007/s10439-010-9901-0

[320] L. Formaggia, A. Moura, and F. Nobile, "On the stability of the coupling of 3D and 1D fluid-structure interaction models for blood flow simulations," *ESAIM Math. Model. Numer. Anal.*, vol. 41, no. 4, pp. 743–769, Jul. 2007, doi: 10.1051/m2an:2007039

[321] J. Janela, A. Moura, and A. Sequeira, "Absorbing boundary conditions for a 3D non-Newtonian fluid–structure interaction model for blood flow in arteries," *Int. J. Eng. Sci.*, vol. 48, no. 11, pp. 1332–1349, Nov. 2010, doi: 10.1016/j.ijengsci.2010.08.004

[322]A. M. Gambaruto, J. Janela, A. Moura, and A. Sequeira, "Sensitivity of hemodynamics in a patient specific cerebral aneurysm to vascular geometry and blood rheology," *Math. Biosci. Eng.*, vol. 8, no. 2, pp. 409–423, 2011, doi: 10.3934/mbe.2011.8.409

[323] A. T. Butt, Y. A. Abakr, and K. B. Mustapha, "Blood flow modelling to improve cardiovascular diagnostics: A preliminary review of 1-D modelling," *Int. J. Eng. Technol.*, vol. 7, no. 4, pp. 25–34, 2018, doi: 10.14419/ijet.v7i4.3.19547

[324] V. C. Rideout, *Mathematical and Computer Modeling of Physiological Systems*, 1991. Prentice Hall.

[325] V. Milišić and A. Quarteroni, "Analysis of lumped parameter models for blood flow simulations and their relation with 1D models," *ESAIM Math. Model. Numer. Anal.*, vol. 38, no. 4, pp. 613–632, Jul. 2004, doi: 10.1051/m2an:2004036

[326] T. Korakiantitis and Y. Shi., "Model Repository. CellML," 2006. http://mod els.cellml.org/exposure/c49d416ae3a5132882e6ea7479ba50f5/ModelMain. cellml/cellml_math (accessed Apr. 29, 2021).

[327] N. Westerhof, F. Bosman, C. J. De Vries, and A. Noordergraaf, "Analog studies of the human systemic arterial tree," *J. Biomech.*, vol. 2, no. 2, pp. 121–143, 1969, doi: 10.1016/0021-9290(69)90024-4

[328] T. J. R. Hughes and J. Lubliner, "On the one-dimensional theory of blood flow in the larger vessels," *Math. Biosci.*, vol. 18, no. 1–2, pp. 161–170, 1973, doi: 10.1016/0025-5564(73)90027-8

[329] M. S. Olufsen, C. S. Peskin, W. Y. Kim, E. M. Pedersen, A. Nadim, and J. Larsen, "Numerical simulation and experimental validation of blood flow in arteries with structured-tree outflow conditions," *Ann. Biomed. Eng.*, vol. 28, no. 11, pp. 1281–1299, 2000, doi: 10.1114/1.1326031

[330] A. S. Olufsen, *Modeling the Arterial System with Reference to an Anesthesia Simulator, 1998*. Roskilde Universitet.

[331] N. Stergiopulos, D. F. Young, and T. R. Rogge, "Computer simulation of arterial flow with applications to arterial and aortic stenoses," *J. Biomech.*, vol. 25, no. 12, pp. 1477–1488, 1992, doi: 10.1016/0021-9290(92)90060-E

[332] J. Lee and N. P. Smith, "Lumped parameter outflow models for 1-D blood flow simulations," *Ann. Biomed. Eng.*, vol. 40, no. 11, pp. 2399–2413, 2012, doi: 10.1007/s10439-012-0583-7

[333] W. E. Bodley, "The non-linearities of arterial blood flow," *Phys. Med. Biol.*, vol. 16, no. 4, pp. 663–672, 1971, doi: 10.1088/0031-9155/16/4/010

[334] V. L. Streeter, W. F. Keitzer, and D. F. Bohr, "Pulsatile pressure and flow through distensible vessels," *Circ. Res.*, vol. 13, pp. 3–20, 1963, doi: 10.1161/01.RES.13.1.3

[335] P. Reymond, F. Merenda, F. Perren, D. Rüfenacht, and N. Stergiopulos, "Validation of a one-dimensional model of the systemic arterial tree," *Am. J. Physiol. Hear. Circ. Physiol.*, vol. 297, no. 1, pp. 208–222, 2009, doi: 10.1152/ajpheart.00037.2009

[336] Q. Pan et al., "A one-dimensional mathematical model for studying the pulsatile flow in microvascular networks," *J. Biomech. Eng.*, vol. 136, no. 1, 2014, doi: 10.1115/1.4025879

[337] Y. H. Sun, T. J. Anderson, K. H. Parker, and J. V. Tyberg, "Wave-intensity analysis: a new approach to coronary hemodynamics," *J. Appl. Physiol.*, vol. 89, no. 4, pp. 1636–1644, 2000. 10.1152/jappl.2000.89.4.1636

[338] E. H. Hollander, G. M. Dobson, J.-J. Wang, K. H. Parker, and J. V. Tyberg, "Direct and series transmission of left atrial pressure perturbations to the pulmonary artery: a study using wave-intensity analysis," *Am. J. Physiol. Circ. Physiol.*, vol. 286, no. 1, pp. H267–H275, Jan. 2004, doi: 10.1152/ajpheart.00505.2002

[339] A. Zambanini, S. L. Cunningham, K. H. Parker, A. W. Khir, S. A. M. G. Thom, and A. D. Hughes, "Wave-energy patterns in carotid, brachial, and radial arteries: A noninvasive approach using wave-intensity analysis," *Am. J. Physiol. – Hear. Circ. Physiol.*, vol. 289, no. 1 58-1, pp. 270–276, 2005, doi: 10.1152/ajpheart.00636.2003

[340] J. M. Harana, Non-invasive, MRI-based calculation of the aortic blood pressure waveform by 0-dimensional flow modelling: Development and testing using in silico and in vivo data. King's College London, 2017. https://kclpure.kcl.ac.uk/portal/en/studentTheses/non-invasive-mri-based-calculation-of-the-aortic-blood-pressure-w

[341] S. Jiang, Z. Q. Zhang, F. Wang, and J. K. Wu, "A personalized-model-based central aortic pressure estimation method," *J. Biomech.*, vol. 49, no. 16, pp. 4098–4106, 2016, doi: 10.1016/j.jbiomech.2016.11.007

[342] M. Khalifé, A. Decoene, F. Caetano, L. de Rochefort, E. Durand, and D. Rodríguez, "Estimating absolute aortic pressure using MRI and a one-dimensional model," *J. Biomech.*, vol. 47, no. 13, pp. 3390–3399, 2014, doi: 10.1016/j.jbiomech.2014.07.018

[343] G. Bárdossy and G. Halász, "A 'backward' calculation method for the estimation of central aortic pressure wave in a 1D arterial model network," *Comput. Fluids*, vol. 73, pp. 134–144, Mar. 2013, doi: 10.1016/j.compfluid.2012.12.014

[344] P. Charlton, M. Aresu, J. Spear, P. Chowienczyk, and J. Alastruey, "Indices to assess aortic stiffness from the finger photoplethysmogram: In silico and in vivo testing," *Artery Res.*, vol. 24, no. C, p. 128, 2018, doi: 10.1016/j.artres.2018.10.217

[345] M. Willemet, P. Chowienczyk, and J. Alastruey, "A database of virtual healthy subjects to assess the accuracy of foot-to-foot pulse wave velocities for estimation of aortic stiffness," pp. 663–675, 2015, doi: 10.1152/ajpheart.00175.2015

[346] S. Vennin et al., "Noninvasive calculation of the aortic blood pressure waveform from the flow velocity waveform: A proof of concept," *Am. J. Physiol. – Hear. Circ. Physiol.*, vol. 309, no. 5, pp. H969–H976, 2015, doi: 10.1152/ajpheart.00152.2015

[347] M. Saito, Y. Ikenaga, M. Matsukawa, Y. Watanabe, T. Asada, and P. Y. Lagrée, "One-dimensional model for propagation of a pressure wave in a model of the human arterial network: Comparison of theoretical and experimental results," *J. Biomech. Eng.*, vol. 133, no. 12, pp. 1–9, 2011, doi: 10.1115/1.4005472

[348] K. H. Parker and C. J. H. Jones, "Forward and backward running waves in the arteries: Analysis using the method of characteristics," *J. Biomech. Eng.*, vol. 112, no. 3, p. 322, 1990, doi: 10.1115/1.2891191

[349] J. J. Wang, A. B. O'Brien, N. G. Shrive, K. H. Parker, and J. V. Tyberg, "Time-domain representation of ventricular-arterial coupling as a windkessel and wave system," *Am. J. Physiol. Hear. Circ. Physiol.*, vol. 284, no. 4 53-4, pp. 1358–1368, 2003, doi: 10.1152/ajpheart.00175.2002

[350] J. J. Wang and K. H. Parker, "Wave propagation in a model of the arterial circulation," *J. Biomech.*, vol. 37, no. 4, pp. 457–470, 2004, doi: 10.1016/j.jbiomech.2003.09.007

[351] B. S. Brook, S. A. E. G. Falle, and T. J. Pedley, "Numerical solutions for unsteady gravity-driven flows in collapsible tubes: Evolution and roll-wave instability of a steady state," *J. Fluid Mech.*, vol. 396, no. May 2014, pp. 223–256, 1999, doi: 10.1017/S0022112099006084

[352] B. S. Brook and T. J. Pedley, "A model for time-dependent flow in (giraffe jugular) veins: Uniform tube properties," *J. Biomech.*, vol. 35, no. 1, pp. 95–107, 2002, doi: 10.1016/S0021-9290(01)00159-2

[353] S. J. Sherwin, V. Franke, J. Peiró, and K. Parker, "One-dimensional modelling of a vascular network in space-time variables," *J. Eng. Math.*, vol. 47, no. 3/4, pp. 217–250, Dec. 2003, doi: 10.1023/B:ENGI.0000007979.32871.e2

[354] D. Bessems, C. G. Giannopapa, M. C. M. Rutten, and F. N. van de Vosse, "Experimental validation of a time-domain-based wave propagation model of blood flow in viscoelastic vessels," *J. Biomech.*, vol. 41, no. 2, pp. 284–291, 2008, doi: 10.1016/j.jbiomech.2007.09.014

[355] L. R. John, "Forward electrical transmission line model of the human arterial system," *Med. Biol. Eng. Comput.*, vol. 42, no. 3, pp. 312–321, May 2004, doi: 10.1007/BF02344705

[356] A. R. Ghigo, J. M. Fullana, and P. Y. Lagrée, "A 2D nonlinear multiring model for blood flow in large elastic arteries," *J. Comput. Phys.*, vol. 350, pp. 136–165, 2017, doi: 10.1016/j.jcp.2017.08.039

[357] S. Boujena, O. Kafi, and N. El Khatib, "A 2D mathematical model of blood flow and its interactions in an atherosclerotic artery," *Math. Model. Nat. Phenom.*, vol. 9, no. 6, pp. 46–68, 2014, doi: 10.1051/mmnp/20149605

[358] A. Lopez-Perez, R. Sebastian, and J. M. Ferrero, "Three-dimensional cardiac computational modelling: Methods, features and applications," *Biomed. Eng. Online*, vol. 14, no. 1, pp. 1–31, 2015, doi: 10.1186/s12938-015-0033-5

[359] X. Xie, M. Zheng, D. Wen, Y. Li, and S. Xie, "A new CFD based non-invasive method for functional diagnosis of coronary stenosis," *Biomed. Eng. Online*, vol. 17, no. 1, pp. 1–13, 2018, doi: 10.1186/s12938-018-0468-6

[360] H. Watanabe, S. Sugiura, H. Kafuku, and T. Hisada, "Multiphysics simulation of left ventricular filling dynamics using fluid-structure interaction finite element method," *Biophys. J.*, vol. 87, no. 3, pp. 2074–2085, 2004, doi: 10.1529/biophysj.103.035840

[361] F. Migliavacca et al., "Multiscale modelling in biofluidynamics: Application to reconstructive paediatric cardiac surgery," *J. Biomech.*, vol. 39, no. 6, pp. 1010–1020, 2006, doi: 10.1016/j.jbiomech.2005.02.021

[362] I. E. Vignon-Clementel, C. Alberto Figueroa, K. E. Jansen, and C. A. Taylor, "Outflow boundary conditions for three-dimensional finite element modeling of blood flow and pressure in arteries," *Comput. Methods Appl. Mech. Eng.*, vol. 195, no. 29–32, pp. 3776–3796, 2006, doi: 10.1016/j.cma.2005.04.014

[363] L. Formaggia, J. F. Gerbeau, F. Nobile, and A. Quarteroni, "On the coupling of 3D and 1D Navier-Stokes equations for flow problems in compliant vessels," *Comput. Methods Appl. Mech. Eng.*, vol. 191, no. 6–7, pp. 561–582, 2001, doi: 10.1016/S0045-7825(01)00302-4

[364] L. Formaggia, A. Quarteroni, and A. Veneziani, "Multiscale models of the vascular system," in *Cardiovascular Mathematics*. Springer, 2009, pp. 395–446.

[365] J. P. Murgo, N. Westerhof, J. P. Giolma, and S. A. Altobelli, "Aortic input impedance in normal man: relationship to pressure wave forms," *Circulation*, vol. 62, no. 1, pp. 105–116, Jul. 1980, doi: 10.1161/01.CIR.62.1.105

[366] S. J. Zieman, V. Melenovsky, and D. A. Kass, "Mechanisms, pathophysiology, and therapy of arterial stiffness," *Arterioscler. Thromb. Vasc. Biol.*, vol. 25, no. 5, pp. 932–943, 2005, doi: 10.1161/01.ATV.0000160548.78317.29

[367] N. Kannathal, U. R. Acharya, E. Y. K. Ng, L. C. Min, J. S. Suri, and J. A. E. Spaan, "Data fusion of multimodal cardiovascular signals," *Adv. Card. Signal Process.*, vol. 1, no. 2, pp. 167–186, 2007, doi: 10.1007/978-3-540-36675-1_6

[368] H. Hall, "A misguided study to test the reliability of traditional Chinese medicine pulse diagnosis," Sciencebasedmedicine.org, 2019. https://scienceba sedmedicine.org/pulse-diagnosis-and-tongue-diagnosis-in-traditional-chin ese-medicine-and-a-misguided-study-to-test-the-reliability-of-pulse-diagno sis/. (accessed Dec. 29, 2019).

[369] B. Williams and P. S. Lacy, "Central aortic pressure and clinical outcomes," *J. Hypertens.*, vol. 27, no. 6, pp. 1123–1125, Jun. 2009, doi: 10.1097/ HJH.0b013e32832b6566

[370] M. J. Roman et al., "Central pressure more strongly relates to vascular disease and outcome than does brachial pressure," *Hypertension*, vol. 50, no. 1, pp. 197–203, Jul. 2007, doi: 10.1161/HYPERTENSIONAHA.107.089078

[371] R. Pini et al., "Central but not brachial blood pressure predicts cardiovascular events in an unselected geriatric population," *J. Am. Coll. Cardiol.*, vol. 51, no. 25, pp. 2432–2439, Jun. 2008, doi: 10.1016/j.jacc.2008.03.031

[372] M. J. Roman, P. M. Okin, J. R. Kizer, E. T. Lee, B. V Howard, and R. B. Devereux, "Relations of central and brachial blood pressure to left ventricular hypertrophy and geometry: the Strong Heart Study," *J. Hypertens.*, vol. 28, no. 2, pp. 384–388, Feb. 2010, doi: 10.1097/HJH.0b013e328333d228

Index

Note: Figures are shown in *italics* and tables in **bold** type. The acronym "CVDs" refers to cardiovascular diseases.

A
Adaptive transfer function (ATF), 32–33
Age, 11, 35, 39, 40
Algorithms, 2, 36, 39, 40, 42, **45**, 55
    backpropagation, 37–38
Angina pectoris, 10
Angiogram, 29
ANNs (artificial neural networks), 37–40
Aortic pressure (PA1), 55
Aortic signals, 55, 59, 60
Aortic valve, 5, 6
Arrhythmia, 12, 38, **43**, **44**
Arterial pressure, 59
Arterial stiffness, 33, 34
Arteries
    coronary, 9, 11, 38
    peripheral, 9, 11, 30–31
    pulmonary, 5, *5*, *6*, 8, 52
Arterioles, 6, 7, 52
Arteriosclerosis, 12, 45
Artificial intelligence, for detection of CVDs, 36–46, **43–45**
Artificial neural networks (ANNs), 37–40
ATF (adaptive transfer function), 32–33
Atheroma, 11
Atrial fibrillation, 40, **43**, **44**
Ayurveda, 20, 23, 24, 60

B
Backpropagation algorithm, 37–38
Biological neural networks, 41
Blood flow, 5–7, *6*, 60, 61
    diminished, 9, 11
    direction of, 22, 47
    models of, **53**
    motion of, 56
    and multiscale models, 57, 58
    and pressure, 33, 57
    in 0D model, 49

Blood pressure (BP), 26
    central, **15–18**, 33, 61
    high, 11, 12, 46
    measurement of, 28–29
Blood vessels, 14, 20, 28, 60
    in cardiovascular system, 4, 6, 9–12
    in cardiovascular system models, 55–58
BP, *see* Blood pressure (BP)
BPro watch, 20

C
CAD (coronary artery disease), 10, 11, 31, 38, **43**
CAP (central aortic pressure), 30–33
Capillary network, 6
Cardiac cycle, 7–8, *8*
Cardiovascular diseases (CVDs)
    artificial intelligence for detection of, 36–46, **43–45**
    central aortic blood pressure waveform for detection of, 30–35, 61
    detection of, 1, 2, 29
    diagnosing of diseases, 23–29, *25*, *27*, *28*
    risk indication for, 35
Cardiovascular risk, 30, 35, 36, 40, 61
Cardiovascular system, 4–12, *5–9*, *11*, 29, 61
Cardiovascular system models, 2, 47–58, **48**, *49*, *50*, **53**, **54**
Central aortic blood pressure waveform, 30–35, 61
Central aortic pressure (CAP), 30–33
Central blood pressure, **15–18**, 33, 61
CHD (coronary heart disease), 8, 9, 12, 40
Chinese pulse diagnosis (CPD), 24, *25*
Cholesterol, 9, 35, 39; high blood, 11, 12
CNN (convolutional neural network), 41, 42–46, *42*, **43–45**
Computational cardiovascular models, **48**
Computational fluid dynamics, 57
Computed tomography (CT) scan, 26, 28

Congenital heart disease, 11, 40
Convolutional neural network (CNN), 41–46, *42*, **43–45**
Coronary artery, 9, 11, 38
Coronary artery disease (CAD), 10, 11, 31, 38, **43**
Coronary heart disease (CHD), 8, 9, 12, 40
CPD (Chinese pulse diagnosis), 24, *25*
CT (computed tomography) scan, 26, 28
CVDs, *see* Cardiovascular diseases (CVDs)

D
Deaths
   due to CVDs, 1, 8–10
   due to hypertension, 40
   major causes of, *9*
   see also Mortality
Deep learning, 41–46, **43–45**
Detection, of CVDs, 1, 2, 29–46, **43–45**, 61
Diabetes, 11, 39
Diagnosing cardiovascular diseases, 23–29, *25*, *27*, *28*
Diagnosis
   Chinese pulse (CPD), 24, *25*
   modern, 25–29, *27*, *28*
   traditional, 23–25, *25*
Diastole, 7, 8, *8*

E
ECG (electrocardiogram), 9, 26, **43–44**
ECG (electrocardiography), 1, 13, 38
ECG electrodes, 26, *27*
ECG signals, *28*, 38, 42, **43**, **44**, 60
Echocardiogram, 26–28
Electrocardiogram (ECG), 9, 26, **43–44**
Electrocardiography (ECG), 1, 13, 38
Endothelial dysfunction, 41
Excess body mass, 11, 39; *see also* Obesity paradox

F
Flexible polymer transistors, 20
Fluid–structure interaction (FSI) model, 47

G
Gender, 11–12, 35, 40
Generalized transfer function (GTF), **16**, 31–34
Genetics, 11, 39
Global Burden of Disease, 8

Global deaths, 1, 8
GTF (generalized transfer function), **16**, 31–34

H
Heart, 4, *5*
   attacks, 9–12, 14, 26, 31, 38, **43**
   conditions, 2, 3, 14, 55, 60–61
   failure, 11, 31, 40, **44**
High blood cholesterol, 11, 12
High blood pressure, 11, 12, 46
Holter monitor, 26, 39
Hypertension, 9, 29–34, 40–41
   pulmonary arterial, 40
   risk for, 32, 34, 46

I
Inferior vena cava (IVC) vein, 5–7
Invasive diagnostic methods, 23, 29, 31, 59
   non-, 23, 29–32, 39, 60, 61
Ischemic heart disease, 9, 10
IVC (inferior vena cava) vein, 5–7

L
Left atrium (LA), *5*, 6–8
Left lungs, *6*
Left ventricle, 6
Left ventricular ejection, 41
Left ventricular pressure (PLV), 55
Lifestyle, 10, 12, 14, 37
Long short-term memory, 42

M
Machine learning, 36–41, *36*, *37*
Magnetic resonance imaging (MRI) scan, 26, 28
Major causes of death, *9*
Medical imaging, 26, 28
Medical technology, 2, 13–22, **15–19**, *19*, *21*, *22*
Modelling, of CVDs, 1, 47–58, **48**, *49*, *50*, **53**, **54**
Modern diagnosis, 25–29, *27*, *28*
Monitoring, 1, 2, 10, *11*, 13–22, **15–19**, *19*, *21*, *22*
Mortality, 1, 8, 10, 11, 29, 61; *see also* Deaths
MPXM2053D piezo-resistive pressure sensor, 20
MRI (magnetic resonance imaging) scan, 26, 28

Multilayer perceptron, 37, *37*
Multiscale models, 57–58
Myocardial infarction, 9–12, 14, 26, 31, 38, **43**

N
Navier–Stokes equations, 47, 55–57
Neural networks, 37
    artificial (ANNs), 37–40
    biological, 41
    recurrent, 42
Noninvasive diagnostic methods, 23, 29–32,
    39, 60, 61
N-point moving average (NPMA), 32, 34

O
Obesity, 11, 39
Obesity paradox, 40
One dimensional (1D) models, 55–57

P
PA1 (aortic pressure), 55
PCG (phonocardiogram), 42, 45, **45**
PDAs (personal digital assistants), 13
Peripheral arteries, 9, 11, 30–31
Peripheral artery disease, 11
Peripheral blood pressure waveform, 61
Personal digital assistants (PDAs), 13
Phonocardiogram (PCG), 42, 45, **45**
Photoelectric sensor, 14, 20–21, *21*, 60
Physical activity, 1, 21, 39
Plaque, 9, 12
PLV (left ventricular pressure), 55
PPV (pulmonary artery pressure), 55
Pressure sensor, 14–20, **15–19**, *19*, 59–60
Primary prevention, 1
PRV (right ventricular pressure), 55
Pulmonary arterial hypertension, 40
Pulmonary artery, 5, *5*, *6*, 8, 52
Pulmonary artery pressure (PPV), 55
Pulmonary valve, *5*, 6
Pulmonary veins, *5*, 6, 8, 52–53
Pulse diagnosis, 24, *25*
Pulse wave signal, 12, 14, 20–22, 31, 59–60

R
RA (right atrium), 5–7, *5*
Radial pulse wave, 14, *19*, 20–22, *22*,
    31, 59–60
Radiofrequency catheter ablation, 38–39
Recurrent neural network, 42

Reynolds number, 47
Right atrium (RA), 5–7, *5*
Right lungs, *6*
Right ventricle (RV), 5–8, *5*
Right ventricular pressure (PRV), 55
Risk detection, 30–46, **43–45**, 61
Risk factors, for CVDs, 1, 9, 11–12, 35, 37,
    39, 40, 61
RV (right ventricle), 5–8, *5*

S
Second systolic pressure of periphery, 33
Sensors
    photoelectric, 14, 20–21, *21*, 60
    pressure, 14–20, **15–19**, *19*
    ultrasonic, 14, 21–22, *22*, 60
Smartphones, 13
Smoking, 1, 9, 11, 35, 39, 40
Stroke, 9, 11, 12, 29, 31, 61
Superior vena cava (SVC) vein, 5–7
Systemic vein, 52–53
Systole, 7, 8, *8*, 33

T
TCM (traditional Chinese medicine),
    23–24, 45
Technology, medical, 2, 13–22, **15–19**,
    19, *21*, *22*
TempR equation, 53, **54**
TempRC equation, 53, **54**
TempRLC equation, 53, **54**
Three dimensional (3D) models, 47, 49, *49*,
    50, 57–59
Traditional Chinese medicine (TCM),
    23–24, 45
Traditional diagnosis, 23–25, *25*
Tricuspid valve, *5*, 6
Tridoshic theory, 24
Two dimensional (2D) models, *49*, 49, 57, 58

U
Ultrasonic sensor, 14, 21–22, *22*, 60
Unhealthy food habits, 1

V
Veins, 4, 6, 7
    inferior vena cava (IVC), 5–7
    narrowing of, 9
    pulmonary, *5*, 6, 8, 52–53
    superior vena cava (SVC), 5–7

systemic, 52–53
vena cava, 5, 8
Vena cava vein, 5, 8

W
Wearable devices, 13–14, 21, 30, 31, 40, 60–61
WHO (World Health Organization), 8
Windkessel model, 53
World Health Organization (WHO), 8

Wrist pulse signal, 12, 14, 24, 25, 60
Wrist radial artery, 60

X
X-ray imaging, 26, 28

Z
Zero dimensional (0D) models, 49–55, *50*, **53**, **54**, 57–59